Quit Smoking (or vaping) in Style

Robert Matthews

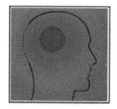

ULTRA CALM LONDON 2017

Quit Smoking (or Vaping) in Style

Copyright © 2017 Robert Matthews

Imprint: Independently published by CreateSpace

ISBN: 9781520946122

AMAZON CREATESPACE

About the author

Robert Matthews has been carrying out quit smoking sessions with phenomenal success since 1996. The success of his method led to the creation of The Quit Smoking Clinic UK in 2001, which has helped people from all walks of life and almost every country in the world to quit, including many well known celebrities. Robert worked for several years in Harley Street, has a degree in Psychology and is a former, part time lecturer at The University of West London.

As a hypnotherapist, he experimented with giving a motivational talk before hypnotising those attending his sessions, claiming that it increased the success rate to almost 100%. Realising that the talk was often enough to make people quit in its own right he decided to share the formula with the world in the form of a book. Robert has three children and lives in London. He is also a musician and actor.

Are YOU in the smoking or vaping trap?

That dark, stinking, scary place they say is so hard to escape from? Looking for the best way out? This book will not only show you were that door to freedom is, it will open that door wider for you than it's ever been opened before. Much wider. That's a promise. I am your escape navigator. Listen carefully to the briefing and you will make it to freedom. I won't push you through that door. I won't even give you a piggy back through the door! Rest assured, however, I will be close at hand. Only you can go through that door. So why wait? When you are ready, let's do it....

Contents

PART FOUR: THE SOLUTION - HOW TO QUIT SMOKING IN STYLE

Foreword

"A cigarette is the perfect type of a perfect pleasure. It is exquisite, and it leaves one unsatisfied. What more can one want?"
- Oscar Wilde

There's only one way to quit smoking...to do it in style!

Smoking is a kind of trap. Once you are in it, it's hard to escape, but every smoker has the power to escape from that trap. That means YOU have the power! If you're the kind of person who likes to do things well - this book is for you. Smoking is a bit like being in a useless relationship and I will show you how can quit smoking just like you would end that relationship.

If on the other hand, you would rather quit in a painful, drawn out, ordinary, low key way, with someone holding your hand for weeks on end - maybe trying to cut down, or using nicotine gum or patches for example, then this book is definitely not for you! After all, according to recent research, nicotine replacement therapy has a failure rate of about 94% (Hillel Alpert 2012).

Quit Smoking in Style basically amounts to a very detailed explanation as to why quitting involves no sacrifice of any kind. It's not a play on words, or some kind of new fangled gimmick. It's not a form of brain washing about the benefits of being a non smoker, nor is it a long winded lecture about how foolish it is to smoke. The main message it contains is that giving up smoking involves NO SACRIFICE from a drug point of view whatsoever. Although smoking (or vaping) can give you pleasure, nicotine is a completely useless drug, and this book will not only tell you why, it will empower you to quit like nothing you have ever heard before, and leave you feeling liberated and wondering why this message is not understood and broadcast by mainstream medicine.

I am convinced that if all smokers understood the message of this book, it would spell the end of smoking and vaping worldwide... forever.

Many people who quit smoking successfully say it was the hardest thing they ever did in their lives. I believe it doesn't have to be that way. They only struggle because they believe they are giving up a useful drug. I am passionate about helping people quit and have been carrying out sessions for over twenty years. I have always had a tremendous amount of success, helping thousands of people, which is the main thing that prompted me to write this book.

Within all of us is a tremendous power, far greater than anything most of us could possibly even begin to imagine. That power may have helped you before in your life, and yet in some areas it may have been blocked. The aim of his book is to summon and release that power through telling you the surprising truth about smoking. Information is power. The goal of this book is to enable anyone to walk free from the smoking trap forever. Words are powerful. The right words can reduce the misery of giving up smoking - or even take it away.

By profession I am a hypnotherapist, but before hypnotising people to stop smoking I always do a motivational talk in order to build up determination to the highest pitch possible. Most of those in my profession know that doing this massively increases the chances of success. Over the years I experimented with the content of the talk, it gradually became longer and longer until eventually I found it had built up my success rate was almost up to 100%. To my amazement, I found that the talk alone was making people quit - even hardened smokers who had tried and failed numerous times were quitting without needing hypnosis! So, I have decided to turn that successful formula into a book, and to share it with the world.

This book is the first, as far as I know, to see the main problem as *nicotine use*, or nicotine addiction, rather than simply smoking. It could easily have been entitled "Quit Nicotine in Style" and addresses nicotine users rather than simply those who obtain the drug through cigarettes. Whether you smoke or vape you are basically a *nicotine user* - in other word a drug user. Smoking and vaping are basically two different forms of nicotine use. It doesn't matter whether you ingest nicotine through smoking, vaping, chewing tobacco, snuff, snus, or through patches and gum - you are a nicotine user. If you experience withdrawal symptoms when you quit - you are almost certainly a nicotine addict. Please don't be alarmed or offended at being called a drug addict. It doesn't mean you lurk in dark alleyways! As you will discover later, learning about the addictive nature of nicotine is key to understanding why the drug can provide no benefit.

This book may also be of comfort to ex-smokers, especially those feeling deprived of the perceived benefits of smoking, who are maybe even contemplating taking up vaping. Sadly, every day, thousands of those who have successfully quit are doing just that, in the false belief that vaping provides a safe, or safer alternative to smoking tobacco. If an ex-smoker takes up vaping they are simply returning into the jaws of nicotine addiction, and, as you read through, you will be left in absolutely no doubt whatsoever, that safe or not, taking nicotine in any form is pointless.

Years ago I was carrying out a quit smoking session when a very heavy smoker told me he believed it would be impossible for him to quit. He was a bit of a character and asked me if I had any special advice for him. Spontaneously I replied, "Smoke in style...quit in style!"

From that day onwards I have always invited people to "Quit Smoking in Style!"

Introduction

Ever wondered how some people, even heavy smokers seem to be able to quit with no effort?

No cutting down, no patches, no gum, no dubious drugs, no complicated list of instructions, no holding on to someone's hand, no hesitation, no apology, no half hearted attempts, no pathetic series of failures?

What is it these people have? Willpower? Wisdom? Intelligence? No, they are just fortunate enough to have the right mindset to quit successfully - they all seem to possess a kind of unshakeable determination. They instinctively realise that the only way to do it is abruptly and permanently...to quit in style. That is the way to minimise or even eliminate withdrawal. This book will share that mindset with you so you can quit smoking (or vaping) with relative ease.

I'm a great believer in individual freedom. If people want to take risks - let them. If people want to take drugs - that's their choice, but once you fully understand why nicotine has no benefit from a drug point of view it will empower you to quit like nothing you have ever heard before. No more cutting down, no more nicotine gum or patches, no more counseling sessions or lectures about how foolish you are. On top of that you won't have even the slightest envy for those people who still smoke or vape!

Why this book is needed

I believe this is a much needed book, because in the United Kingdom one in five adults (10 million people) still smoke, and most of them have tried to quit at some point, often numerous times. In the USA there are about 40 million smokers. In fact smoking is increasing in the developing world at such a rate that a third of the world's adult population now smoke! In China there are now 358 million smokers - incredibly, that's more people than there are living in the whole of the US!

Research suggests that the average smoker who started in their teens will have made over 20 failed attempts to quit by the time they are forty (Borland 2011). This means there is a lot of unsuccessful quitting going on! The overall rate of quitting success has barely increased in the last twenty years, suggesting that nicotine replacement, other quit smoking drugs, and counseling has had little or no effect.

I realise there have been books about the uselessness of smoking and vaping before, but with millions still puffing away worldwide, the message has obviously missed the mark or is just not being understood. I believe it's because the message was flawed. There is a much needed, clearer, and more memorable explanation.

The notion that nicotine is pointless as a recreational drug was first put forward in the 1950s by the Scottish physician Lennox Johnston. It was then broadcast more widely by the quit smoking guru Allen Carr in 1985, but there were flaws in both of their approaches. Large chunks of the jigsaw were still missing, and I believe this is why the truth about nicotine failed to become generally understood or accepted, both by the public and health organisations. Not only that, the scientific community has never adopted the message. Confusingly, Carr told smokers that the pleasure of smoking was an illusion! He also demonised the part of the mind or body that craves nicotine calling it the "Nicotine Monster". Furthermore, he believed adamantly that informing smokers of the dangers of smoking was unhelpful and would not help them quit. *Quit smoking in Style* is a radical change from all that. Firstly, it doesn't hide the dangers from you. It reveals the horrific truth about smoking in all its terrifying detail, explaining why smoking (or vaping) is not only slowly killing you, it is damaging your body, sapping your strength, reducing your energy, lowering your sex drive, and aging you with every puff.

Secondly, you are not repeatedly told that the pleasure is an illusion - of course there is a pleasure! Why else would anyone smoke? Saying it is an illusion is like telling people to deny their own senses, or experience. If there were no pleasure, why would people find it so hard to quit?

Instead of denying the pleasure, *Quit Smoking in Style* explains how the pleasure comes purely from relieving nicotine withdrawal - which can be a great pleasure. It takes a far more scientific look at nicotine, in an attempt to establish once and for all - without any doubt - that there is no benefit to smoking or vaping. With so many people still smoking, and millions more starting up every year, the message is obviously not being understood. Coming as it does from a different angle, this book provides a much needed, clearer explanation as to why smoking or vaping has no benefit.

Thirdly, there is no denial you will need willpower to succeed. It doesn't tell you you won't need determination. Some authors claim that if you follow their methods properly there will be no withdrawal symptoms at all when you quit. Promises like this simply get people down when the fairytale doesn't happen and they sink further into the nicotine trap. Nicotine is an addictive drug so of course there is usually withdrawal. Instead, Q*uit Smoking in Style* aims to steadily build up your willpower into an unstoppable force! The book's realistic aim is to minimise withdrawal and make quitting more like a walk in the park.

I believe the way to empower people is by telling them the truth. For the first time, you are told the *whole truth* about smoking - how the choice of tobacco was a tragic mistake of history, why smoking is statistically more dangerous than fighting in World War One, and above all, why the drug nicotine has absolutely no benefit to any human being.

Incidentally, there is no "Nicotine Monster" inside you! Believing there is a negative force within you to do battle against is unhelpful. Cravings arise automatically from the autonomic nervous system. It's as if there is a computer inside the brain that doesn't realise you've quit or that nicotine is useless and unnecessary. If it produces a craving for nicotine it, ironically, only trying to help.

You will be told the fascinating story of how the world came to smoke in the first place. Again, the history of smoking is ignored by most writers, but I believe the more knowledge you have, the easier it is to quit. People often regard smoking as natural, but you may be surprised to learn that the white man only "discovered" tobacco in 1492, which is little more than 500 years ago. You will be able to decide for yourself whether Christopher Columbus's crew really knew what they were doing when they chose to bring back tobacco from the Native American Indians in 1493.

Most of the time the natives did not even inhale the smoke. Learning how little we knew about smoking and other drugs compared to the ancient wisdom of the Native Americans is extremely eye opening. The Europeans couldn't even keep tobacco alight, so they added potassium nitrate (the same chemical that makes gunpowder and sparklers burn) to the tobacco mixture. It is still added to cigarettes! I believe it's worth knowing about things like that.

The book also uncovers a number of other widespread myths about smoking. For example did you know that only about one fifth of smoking related deaths are actually caused by lung cancer? Yes, that's right, only one fifth. Younger smokers are often oblivious to the more immediate dangers of smoking - how even an occasional cigarette or vape can mutate cells in the mouth, throat, larynx or esophagus leading to cancer. Not only that, but as long as you still smoke there will never be a single day in your life when you are at your full potential physically or looks wise - even if you are just an occasional smoker.

Another myth is that most of the withdrawal symptoms are physical. In actual fact the physical withdrawal is very mild - it's the psychological withdrawal, the dreadful feeling of being deprived, the false assumption you have given up a useful drug, that makes withdrawal pangs so much unbearable for many people.

You will hear the full truth about smoking, written by somebody who was once a 20 a day smoker and who since quitting has been working at the sharp end, as a quit smoking specialist for over twenty years. If you are finding it difficult to stop or are experiencing withdrawal symptoms this is the book for you. If you are looking for a magic bullet to help you handle cravings, this is the nearest thing you will find on the planet. You'll learn of the false assumptions about smoking that are deeply rooted in the minds of so many of us. The way you think and feel about nicotine can have a massive effect on the severity and degree of any withdrawal, if any, you experience.

You will soon notice that this book is packed with metaphors, analogies and stories. Anyone who has ever studied Neuro Linguistic Programming (NLP) will know how powerful metaphor can be. As a hypnotherapist I am very aware of the power it has over the mind and body. It is a surprisingly effective and rapid way of "reprogramming" the brain without using formal hypnosis. Metaphor helps get messages across and also changes how we think and feel. It's use was popularised by the American Milton Erickson, the most influential hypnotherapist of all time.

Many colleagues, friends and clients have encouraged me to share this knowledge with the world. So here it is. It's a big book but then smoking is a big problem. You don't need a nanny to hold your hand when you quit or learn a set of complicated instructions to remember all day long. Once you truly understand the message of this book it will enable you not just to quit but...quit in style!

Part One
Why Nicotine is Useless

1- The Nicotine Delusion

Clearly when someone smokes they feel pleasure or relief - so how can it be useless? Why else would anyone smoke? Why else would anyone vape? How can anyone deny that there is a pleasure to be found in taking in a long, satisfying drag of cigarette smoke from time to time?

You might have previously heard people claiming that smoking has no benefit, and there are many people (smokers, non smokers, or ex. smokers alike) who pay lip service to the notion - but the majority of us simply don't see how it can be true. Most people would agree that smoking for the most part is habit forming and extremely risky...but surely if you take that risk, in return you get to enjoy some kind of pleasant feeling from the drug nicotine? Isn't that obvious and undeniable?

The main message of his book can be put into one, simple sentence:

"Taking nicotine is pointless - it is not the drug itself that brings about any pleasure - one hundred percent of the pleasure from smoking or vaping comes from relieving the withdrawal symptoms for nicotine that crop up between each cigarette or dose."

Most of this book is dedicated to backing up that statement by providing enough detail and evidence to convince even the most hardened skeptic that smoking is a pointless trap and that nicotine is the world's most useless recreational drug.

Some of you might think that saying nicotine has no benefit as a drug is ridiculous. How can that possibly be true? How can anyone suggest the drug is useless when clearly, throughout our entire lives, since being small children, we have witnessed the pleasure and relief it gives to people who smoke? Many of us have experienced the pleasure for ourselves, we have enjoyed the lift, the temporary high, are loathe to stop smoking or vaping and miss out on all the benefits and comfort from the drug. After all, why would it be so hard for many people to quit if it were useless? If this message were true, surely quit smoking organisations, doctors and scientists would broadcast it?

And yet, incredibly...it's true!

You see, from a pharmacological point of view, nicotine is 100% a stimulant drug. It cannot relax you, give you a lift, or give you any euphoric experience at all unless you have become hooked on it. The real pleasure or "kick" from smoking comes entirely from the pleasurable experience of eliminating the withdrawal symptoms of nicotine which build up between each and every cigarette. In other words it is the pleasure of returning to normal, returning to the level that non smokers are experiencing the whole time. Ironically, the stimulant effect of nicotine, though mild, does the opposite to relax you!

To put it another way, the pleasure of smoking, though real, isn't coming from the drug itself. *It is the brain rewarding you for replenishing the drug*, which is something totally different. Nicotine can't relax you, which is why, paradoxically, the drug is totally useless.

You don't have to give up smoking or vaping to experience withdrawal symptoms for nicotine - they crop up in between each cigarette. The drug leaves the body very quickly and within half an hour or so of stubbing out a cigarette, or finishing a vape, most of it has been excreted. The body must do this because the substance is so toxic it will result in death unless removed. Almost as soon as nicotine levels begin to fall, withdrawal symptoms begin.

The first niggle or desire for the next cigarette is a result of the brain or body calling for more nicotine as levels drop. The smoker may find themselves less able to enjoy whatever activity they are engaged in. As time goes by and nicotine levels drop further, there is an increasing desire to smoke. Heavy smokers, who are much more deeply addicted, experience the withdrawal most quickly, often within minutes of finishing the previous cigarette. Lighter or occasional smokers may be free from withdrawal for considerably longer, sometimes even days, but eventually the withdrawal symptoms begin to take the edge off their enjoyment of life and the need to smoke becomes more urgent.

If ignored, the desire to smoke will gradually develop into a stronger desire and then eventually a longing or craving. At some stage, the smoker gives in and smokes another cigarette, thus relieving the withdrawal symptoms. However, each new cigarette then re-addicts the smoker, the fresh dose of nicotine begins to leave the body again, and therefore the cycle continues. Most smokers are not aware that all this is going on in between cigarettes or vapes. They are unaware that the gradually increasing desire to smoke again and the unpleasant feelings of being tense, anxious, incomplete or lacking in confidence are due to nicotine withdrawal. As nicotine levels drop, the smoker begins to feel unable to concentrate as easily, may feel stressed, irritable, empty or just in need of relief. Most smokers have no idea that the desire to smoke the next cigarette is the desire to come out of withdrawal or keep the withdrawal symptoms at bay. Instead they presume that they are in the *habit* of enjoying a regular lift, or that they are stressed by life and that the desire to smoke, or for nicotine, is the desire to enjoy a useful drug that will help them relax.

The irony is that NONE of the pleasure of smoking comes from the drug nicotine. This cannot be stressed enough. ALL of the pleasure comes from relieving the withdrawal symptoms for the drug, which crop up between each nicotine dose. As those withdrawal symptoms are eliminated the smoker rises up to the level a non smoker is experiencing all the time. This is because non smokers never have withdrawal symptoms for nicotine. They are at the top level all day long. In fact, nicotine as a drug is incapable of relaxing anyone. When those withdrawal symptoms are relived or removed the smoker has the sensation of returning to normal. That may not sound very exciting but returning to normal can be a huge pleasure - like hanging upside down and then returning to your feet. It can be an incredible feeling of relief or pleasure. Whilst the smoker is enjoying the feeling of relief, the stimulant effect of nicotine is working simultaneously in the background, but the effect is so mild it is not usually noticeable at all. In fact it raises the blood pressure, increases heart rate, raises metabolism - the very opposite to relaxation or sedation.

For almost five hundred years the human race has made the false assumption that tobacco, although dangerous, contains a drug capable of giving pleasure, relaxation and other benefits. An assumption that rivals the flat earth theory in terms of its inaccuracy. One day, we will marvel at how long it was before we worked out the truth. As with any paradigm shift it can take a little time before the truth sinks in. This is not surprising because it goes against the grain of everything you have believed or assumed about smoking and nicotine your entire life.

It means that every smoker out there is smoking for nothing. It means that both smoking and vaping are pointless. Sadly, most of those who smoke or vape have absolutely no idea that this is so.

The first person to put forward the idea that smoking was pointless from a drug point of view was the Scottish physician and author Lennox Johnston in his book "The Disease of Tobacco Smoking and it's Cure" (1957) when he made the claim:

"No smoker derives positive pleasure and benefit from tobacco. The bliss of headache or toothache relieved is analogous to that of craving for tobacco appeased."

Johnson was way ahead of his time with such a revolutionary statement but was ignored and even shunned by the medical establishment, many of whom smoked pipes and cigarettes whilst they worked! It was also at a time when virtually all adults smoked and smoking was considered by most to be a harmless habit.

The message was later reinforced by the quit smoking author Allen Carr in his 1985 book "The Easy way to Quit Smoking" although it is quite possible that Carr came to the same conclusion independently. The belief that nicotine is a useless drug is shared by Johnston, Carr and myself, although, as I have already mentioned, Carr's message about smoking differs fundamentally to my own in many ways. Anyone who has read his book and failed to quit may find it useful to read about these differences, which are outlined in a later chapter.

The hallmark of an accurate theory is that it can be verified, not just from one, but from several different angles, and as you read on you will be provided with abundant evidence and left in no doubt whatsoever that by quitting smoking you are giving up nothing. If the truth has not already hit you right between the eyes - when it does it is a eureka moment! That moment, when the full implications of this message become clear can be very liberating, as all the pieces of the smoking trap fall into place. When I carry out quit smoking sessions I often notice that some people, especially those who are heavily addicted or have previously found it difficult to quit, cannot help but smile with relief as they finally understand why smoking truly is useless and that by becoming a non smoker they are giving up nothing from a drug point of view....whatsoever.

This book is nothing if not thorough! The message that nicotine use is pointless and why it is pointless is repeated dozens of times, in different ways and from an assortment of different angles. Please forgive the repetition if you have already made the breakthrough. However, I would advise you to keep reading to make sure you have no doubt whatsoever and that the truth is permanently embedded in your mind.

2 - The Paracetamol addict

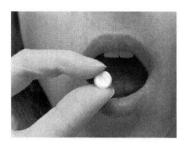

Being hooked on nicotine is as useless as being hooked on Paracetamol.

The uselessness of nicotine can be illustrated by looking at how people hooked on Paracetamol get pleasure from the drug. Paracetamol in itself cannot give pleasure - it is just an over the counter painkiller. You can verify this for yourself very easily by trying one on an occasion when you're not in pain. Like the nicotine addict, the pleasure a Paracetamol addict receives when they take one, come solely from coming out of withdrawal for the drug.

Many over the counter drugs such as painkillers, cough medicines and motion sickness pills can become addictive if taken for lengthy periods. In the UK, thousands of people become hooked on drugs such as Paracetamol when suffering from chronic pain such as tension headaches, nerve pain, back pain or period pains. Well known examples of this are Nurofen and Paracetamol. The late comedian Mel Smith famously became addicted to Nurofen Plus when he was suffering from pain caused by gout. At one point he was taking up to 50 tablets a day, and in retrospect he said:

"I didn't dare tell a soul. Like an alcoholic hiding his bottles...*they just helped me relax*"

Relax? How can a painkiller help someone relax?

Imagine the following scenario:

A young woman hurts her back and develops chronic back pain. She decides to take Paracetamol for its mild analgesic effects, and finds that taking several tables a day keeps the pain under control. She continues on this dose for many weeks, not realising it is possible to become hooked on the drug. After a couple of months her back heals and the pain goes away for good, but she realises she now has a new problem. If she stops taking her regular daily dose of Paracetamol she finds she feels anxious, nervous and irritable. She visits her doctor who realises she has become hooked on the drug. She is informed that the anxiousness and irritability are actually withdrawal symptoms from Paracetamol.

On returning home she attempts to stop taking the drug but when she does the withdrawal symptoms soon become unbearable. There is no pain anywhere in her body yet she has a craving for the painkiller. She opens the bottle of Paracetamol and takes another one. The fresh dose begins to bring her out of withdrawal surprisingly quickly and all the withdrawal symptoms of anxiety and irritability disappear. She feels lifted, incredibly euphoric and relaxed. It is a wonderful sensation as all the anxiety evaporates, she feels calm as all the stress goes and she returns to her normal state. For a while the amount of Paracetamol in her body is high, and she continues to feel relaxed but over the next four hours it is steadily excreted from her body. As this happens the withdrawal symptoms steadily return. Over time they deepen until she is back in the same state of anxiety and tension she had temporarily escaped from.

Unable to bear it she returns to the bottle and decides to take another tablet, even though she knows that doing this will re-addict her. As she removes the cap from the bottle she is already lifted by a feeling of anticipation, thinking of the pleasure of coming out of withdrawal again. As she swallows the pill she notices the familiar taste she once found bitter and unpleasant, is now something she is growing to like. This is because she has begun to associate the taste with the pleasure of coming out of withdrawal - a kind of conditioning. As the drug is absorbed a blissful feeling of relief fills all of her body and mind. She is well and truly hooked.

Each time she takes another tablet she escapes from withdrawal, but each tablet re-addicts her. She longs to escape from the cycle but cannot face enduring the withdrawal...and the miserable cycle goes on. She is in a trap. And there is worse to come. After a few weeks she finds she has to take a higher, more frequent dose in order to come fully out of withdrawal. Eventually she limits herself to twenty Paracetamol a day.

Of course it is not the pain killing, analgesic effect of the drug that is relaxing her and giving her pleasure each time she takes it. It is the elimination of drug withdrawal - the reversal of the tension and irritability that accumulate as Paracetamol is excreted from the body. Paracetamol is simply a pain killer. She is not taking the drug because she is in pain, therefore the drug itself is useless to her. She is now a slave to a drug that cannot even relax her. As mentioned earlier, any pain free person taking Paracetamol as an experiment will testify to the fact that it does not provide any freedom from anxiety or stress. It is not capable of providing a lift, a high or any positive feeling whatsoever. Pleasure can only be obtained by being hooked on the drug and coming out of withdrawal.

By becoming hooked on nicotine you are in a very similar situation. Like Paracetamol, nicotine cannot relax you. It is actually just a mild stimulant, incapable of relaxing anyone, unless you become hooked on it in the same way that people become hooked on Paracetamol. This is why the first cigarette provides no pleasure from a drug point of view. All you are receiving is the very mild stimulant effect from nicotine, such as a slight increase in blood pressure. Such affects are not pleasurable and are barely noticeable. Over The Counter drugs like Paracetamol show how it is possible to become hooked on a drugs that are completely useless from a recreational point of view.

As far as I know, no one has ever deliberately taken a regular dose of Paracetamol in order to become hooked, but if they succeeded, they too would be able to take the tablets, say twenty times a day and enjoy the pleasurable sensation of eliminating withdrawal symptoms each time. Why would anybody do that? That would simply make life more stressful as they would be spending most of the day in different stages of withdrawal. Why would anyone deliberately become hooked on a drug incapable of give a feeling of relaxation or pleasure, capable only of incapable of alleviating pain?

But just imagine for a moment that you deliberately become hooked on Paracetamol. Once this is achieved, you experiment and find that taking say, 20 tablets a day, keeps the cravings away. You are in control of when you take each tablet, in other words you decide where and when to come out of withdrawal. In between each tablet you slowly go into withdrawal, but on taking the next one you enjoy the sublime pleasure of coming out. You begin to swear by them, and people witnessing the pleasure you experience when coming out of withdrawal assume that somehow the drug has a paradoxical dual action. It can be a pain killer one minute and provide an undeniable lift the next. Soon friends and work colleagues follow your lead and deliberately become hooked on Paracetamol. They even give them the endearing nickname, "Pannies", reminiscent of how people affectionately refer to cigarettes as "Ciggies" or call rollups as "Rollies".

Soon Pannies are all the rage. People find taking them in the car helps make driving more bearable. They appear to help you concentrate, help solve problems, help with boredom, nerves and stress. People take bottles of Pannies to work, nipping outside every now and then for a Pannie break. They go down well on social occasions when there is a group of Pannie users, and of course, there's nothing quite like a Pannie with a drink, or the "after Pannie." The first Pannie of the day seems to be the most pleasurable, because overnight you go without a Paracetamol for the longest period of time, and therefore wake up experiencing he deepest withdrawal of the twenty four hour cycle.

Of course there is no benefit whatsoever from being hooked on Paracetamol. What I have described is nothing more than a terrible trap, a ridiculous trap. Getting hooked on any drug is bad enough, but getting hooked on a drug that cannot relax you or give you anything whatsoever is totally and utterly pointless. That's more or less exactly what happens when you become hooked on nicotine, you become a slave to a completely useless and mild stimulant drug that is just as incapable of relaxing you as Paracetamol.

Hopefully by now you will have a clearer picture as to why nicotine addiction is equally pointless. The best way out of Paracetamol addiction is to throw all the tablets or capsules into the bin, and never touch them again, knowing that by doing this, that you are escaping from a trap and that there is no sacrifice being made from a drug point of view whatsoever. Remember, when you quit smoking you are also making no sacrifice. In fact you are escaping from the most useless, pointless and destructive recreational drug on the planet.

3 - Addiction denial

Despite listening to this argument, some smokers, especially light smokers, do not truly believe that they are drug addicts in the first place. They don't like being put into the same category as people who inject themselves with needles in back alleyways - so they deny that nicotine is an addictive drug. They believe that they smoke through choice, rather than through addiction. This may be the case with the odd occasional smoker, but all other smokers, whether they realise it or not, are lighting up or vaping, in order to relieve withdrawal pangs. If you are in any doubt, the main question to ask yourself is, if smoking is simply a habit, why is it that so many smokers can't stop even when they know cigarettes are killing them?

It doesn't help that there is no scientifically accepted definition of addiction. Dictionaries definitions are surprisingly vague, for example The Cambridge Dictionary describes addiction as:

"The need or strong desire to do or to have something, or a very strong liking for something"

Just a need or strong desire? Considering there is so much debate about whether certain substances are addictive or not, you'd expect there to a far clearer definition. I believe a substance is addictive if people experience unpleasant withdrawal symptoms or cravings when they attempt to stop taking it. Judged by this standard, nicotine is clearly addictive because when attempting to quit (usually through fear of fatal illnesses) so many smokers fail. The fact that some smokers are unable to stop even after undergoing surgery for life threatening illnesses caused by smoking, also demonstrates how addictive nicotine is. However, many of those who find it hard to quit give reasons other than the drug addiction, saying, for example, that cigarettes give them a indispensable "plus", or that they give them something to do with their hands.

The hands one is easy to disprove. If smokers are given herbal cigarettes as a substitute when they quit they have plenty to do with their hands, but typically after smoking the first packet they stop, saying they find them unsatisfying...because they contain no nicotine!

Sometimes a nicotine addict will do anything for a cigarette. Prisoners of war in World War Two camps would swap their food rations in order to get a cigarette - which meant going hungry - rather than go without a cigarette. Was that because of habit?

No substance known to mankind is consumed on a daily basis with such frequency as cigarettes - more frequently even than food.

The notion that smoking is purely a habit

Despite all this, the notion that smoking is a habit still persists. Armed by the lack of a general consensus as to what amounts to an addiction, many smokers continue to insist that they smoke purely because they are seeking pleasure, rather than being forced to smoke in order to relieve symptoms of drug withdrawal. If they smoke twenty a day, for example, they claim that this is entirely through choice. When asked why they feel the need to smoke so many cigarettes every day they usually say it is because they find them enjoyable, they provide a useful boost or a helpful crutch. Asked why they do not quit, they typically say that they find it difficult to break such an enjoyable and useful habit!

This view that smoking is a habit is hardly surprising when you consider that both the tobacco industry and the medical profession almost universally denied that nicotine was an addictive drug until well into the Twentieth Century. Prior to the lung cancer scare of the 1960s few smokers ever bothered even attempt to quit. With so few people quitting or even wanting to quit in those days, the difficulties encountered were little known, so it isn't surprising that smoking was looked upon as being a vice or habit. During the 1960s however, a growing number of smokers became fearful of the health consequences and eventually, the majority were expressing the desire to stop... yet they were failing to do so. With so many smokers desperate to quit and unable to do so how could there any longer be any doubt that nicotine was addictive?

Lennox Johnston, the Scottish physician, was the first person to carry out research into the addictive nature of nicotine. He injected a group of smokers with nicotine, and soon many of them preferred the injections they were given to smoking cigarettes. He concluded that:

"Smoking tobacco is essentially a means of administering nicotine, just as smoking opium is a means of administering morphine."

Finally, when nicotine replacement therapy became common in the 1990s the addictive nature of nicotine became clear. It was thought that putting smokers on nicotine patches would reduce motivation to smoke by getting smokers out of the "habit" of lighting up cigarettes at strategic points of the day, but in over 90% of cases it failed. Typically they would indeed get out of the habit of lighting up cigarettes for weeks on end only to return to them soon after the patch was removed and the nicotine supply ended.

Not only that, it was found that some people trying to free themselves from smoking became hooked on nicotine gum or patches! After this it became virtually impossible to deny that nicotine was addictive.

Cutting down never works

If smoking were purely a habit then heavy smokers would be able to successfully cut down and become light smokers. In the course of my job I have never met a smoker who was able to do this. Almost every heavy smoker has tried at some stage, to cut down and become a light or occasional smoker and absolutely every one of them has failed. People don't realise that being a nicotine addict is just like being an alcoholic. Everybody knows that once an alcoholic quits they can't even take a sip - or they will go back to drinking. If they try just having one they are back on the slippery slope and will gradually end up drinking whatever amount they were used to before - without exception. It's exactly the same with smoking - it's a one way street.

The Plan

Many smokers eventually manage to quit and go several months or a year without cigarettes or nicotine, only to try having the occasional cigarette in an attempt to re-invent themselves as an occasional smoker. They frequently decide to do this spontaneously, when having a few drinks on holiday, for example, or when in the company of someone who has only ever been a light smoker. The ex-smoker typically envies those who still smoke, especially occasional smokers, and decides to risk having one, usually as part of a plan to return to smoking and become an occasional smoker themselves.

I call this "The Plan." The Plan is very appealing to smokers and is based on the notion that smoking is purely a habit. The logic being, that once they are no longer in the "habit" of smoking, say 20 a day, they can then return to smoking, perhaps after a year or so and just have the odd cigarette or puff. Almost every heavy smoker has tried re-inventing themselves as an occasional smoker at some stage.

The Plan always fails. It fails in 100% of cases. There are absolutely no exceptions whatsoever. This is because when you smoke you are a nicotine addict, just as surely as someone who takes heroin is a heroin addict. If you have another dose you will simply re-addict yourself and then slide down the slippery slope back to where you started. Addiction does not fade with the passage of time.

Every day, somewhere in the world, thousands of people try "The Plan", encouraged by the notion that smoking is basically a habit and also because the fact that nicotine is an extremely addictive drug is not broadcast by the mainstream media. Every single one of them will eventually return to smoking as many cigarettes as they did before.

Even now, in The Twenty First Century, the message that nicotine is addictive is glossed over or barely mentioned by doctors or health organisations, and addiction denial is therefore still widespread. In all the years that I have conducted quit smoking sessions almost every single person attending those sessions refers to smoking as a habit, failing to mention the word addiction. This is a great shame because understanding the addictive nature of nicotine is key to understanding why smoking is a trap and why quitting, rather than giving anything up, is an escape from that trap.

In order to appreciate that smoking is an addiction it is helpful to look at how we get into the smoking trap in the first place. Smoking always begins as a choice, but the main thing to keep in mind here is that no one, absolutely no one deliberately goes on to become a regular or heavy smoker. Nobody wakes up one day and says to themselves "from now on I will smoke all day, every day from morning till night". It happens gradually because nicotine is addictive.

4 - How we are drawn into the nicotine trap

The image of smoking can be alluring or glamorous...if you are in any doubt just look at the front cover of this book!

Ironically, it's not the drug that draws us in the first place. Virtually no one starts smoking because they are seeking out a useful drug. Almost everyone starts for two reasons, firstly, the desire to bond with those who already smoke, and secondly the lure of the image of smoking. Almost all of us are attracted to the image of smoking at some time in our lives! We want to look and feel worldly, mature, confident and in control...or even glamorous. To the adolescent, smoking is a bridge to the adult world, and speaks of self assurance or rebellion.

For decades, movie and TV stars would typically handle difficult situations by lighting up a cigarette. They would reflect on things coolly and patiently, surrounded by a sophisticated halo of smoke, whilst the non smokers looked on in a helpless state of tension.

I haven't touched a cigarette for many years now, but I remember when I started smoking as a teenager. It was the image that drew me in - it made me feel like a bit of a rebel and came with a readymade identity and set of mannerisms and poses. Most of the males in my circle of friends smoked, and those who didn't were considered to be "wet." Not only that but being a non smoker was sending out all the wrong signals to fun loving, rule breaking girls - the kind that every hot blooded young male was after. All of those girls seemed to smoke, and if you turned down a cigarette you were put into the dreaded "nice guy" bracket.

As soon as I started smoking it seemed to open up a whole new world to me. It appeared that most of the open minded, interesting, and glamorous people smoked. The fact it was risky didn't really bother me because I was young and felt immortal. Not only that, it gave me the ability to look super relaxed whenever I chose and also was a great way to interact socially. It seemed to give me confidence and style and I loved it.

When I quit years later, the loss of the image didn't bother me at all it - it was the loss of what I regarded to be a useful drug, an essential crutch that was so difficult. It was like parting with a helpful, albeit dangerous friend. Giving up was a drawn out, painful sacrifice, and I envied those who still smoked. That envy went on for years.

These days, I wouldn't smoke even if there was a safe cigarette! It's not that I'm anti drug or being politically correct, it's just that when you fully understand why nicotine is the world's most useless recreational drug, and that it can do nothing for you, you will feel the same.

Be wary of anyone who tells you there are no social benefits to smoking - because it is the very reason most of us start. However, when you quit, it is likely the image of the smoker has now become a negative one and these days you are feeling more like a social leper. Regardless as to whether the image, or social benefit of smoking still has any value to you or not, when you quit you can celebrate that you are not only walking away from something that brings illness and death, but also from a drug that has no benefit of any kind.

The first cigarette

"When you give people nicotine for the first time, most people don't like it. It's different from many other addictive drugs, for which most people say they enjoy the first experience and would try it again."

(Roland Griffiths, professor of psychiatry and behavioral sciences at the Johns Hopkins University School)

Having the first cigarette can be as exciting as joining the army. A bit like joining a band of fearless, worldly, risk takers. You now live for the moment, live life to the full and to hell with all those hypocritical ex-smokers who tell you to avoid the natural pleasures of life!

But if anyone starts smoking hoping to find pleasure or satisfaction from a drug point of view then they are going to find that first cigarette very disappointing...even puzzling. As I shall repeat many times in this book, the pleasure of smoking can only come once you're hooked because it arises entirely from relieving the withdrawal symptoms of nicotine - which are of course absent when we have that first puff. The act of doing something rebellious or forbidden may have been exhilarating...but as far as a pleasurable effect from a drug point of view...nothing.

If you ask people to recall their first ever experience of inhaling tobacco smoke, almost everyone who remembers it reports feelings of nausea, light headedness or at the very least being unable to take more than a few puffs. If you then ask if they noticed any pleasant effect from a drug point of view, they almost unanimously say no!

This complete lack of drug induced pleasure is usually a little puzzling for the first time smoker, especially if they observe more experienced smokers around clearly getting considerable pleasure from the same brand of cigarette. Some make the false assumption it is the very noticeable light headed feeling, or even a bodily feeling of heaviness that others are finding so pleasurable. In fact, experienced smokers barely notice those things because they become accustomed to them. The light headed feeling is simply caused by the temporary buildup of carbon dioxide in the blood.

The first time smoker is surprised anyone could ever become hooked on cigarettes seeing as they can detect no pleasure from the drug whatsoever. In the unlikely event that they own up to this, they may be given reassurances from their more experienced peers that you need to persist with smoking before you notice the pleasure, but even so, the first timer is usually convinced that they will never, ever, become hooked on cigarettes.

Try and recall the first time you inhaled. You may or may not have experienced nausea or other well known unpleasant side effects of the first cigarette, but most likely you were expecting to detect some kind of pleasure from the drug nicotine. Unless you were already hooked through passive smoking or possible smoking spliffs, this will have been impossible. Nicotine is a stimulant drug that provides no lift, rush, or pleasure from the first ever dose. In itself, it never provides any pleasure at all.

The first encounter with alcohol is noticeably different. If you give a child a sufficient quantity of cider, wine or beer, for example, it will certainly notice the intoxicating effects - right from the first dose. The same goes for the first dose of cocaine, heroin, in fact just about any recreational drug...except nicotine.

The Trap

When we start smoking, at whatever age, for a short time we are in control and smoke purely out of choice. The absence of drug pleasure from the very first cigarette encourages us to believe we will never become dependent or addicted. It leads us to conclude that if we wanted to we'd be able to quit without any trouble. This is why so many of us go on to become occasional smokers, and we accept further cigarettes for the same reason we had the first one - for the bonding, the kudos, the worldliness, the excitement, or just because it is a good social prop. We enjoy the posing, though subsequent cigarettes are still hard to tolerate and smoked cautiously and slowly. However, despite delivering no pleasure nicotine is very quickly addictive, and the majority of people who persist with smoking soon notice they *are* beginning to get a pleasure. This is the pleasure of relieving the withdrawal symptoms that are now accruing between each cigarette. For most, it's the start of a slippery slope. The brain demands more and more nicotine, the withdrawal between cigarettes comes on more rapidly and becomes deeper. The smoker is trapped.

Choice has now gone, things are out of our control, almost as if the smoker is now programmed to smoke, as if there is a computer in the brain which is now in control, not just of the desire to smoke, but also where and when this occurs. Eventually the smoker has to smoke just to kill the craving, starting from first thing in the morning. This was never the plan, this was not what they wanted to end up doing! At this stage, if the smoker attempts to go for an extended time without smoking they find they simply cannot do it without craving nicotine, so they give in and smoke at intervals all day long. The smoker is now a slave to a drug that cannot relax or give pleasure.

The average smoker eventually limits themselves to a packet a day, unless alcohol interferes with their normal self control, in which case they will likely smoke considerably more. At night the cycle is interrupted by sleep, meaning that on awakening next day the regular smoker has gone much deeper into withdrawal than can occur if they smoke at regular intervals during the day. The first cigarette of the day is therefore, generally experienced as being the most pleasurable because the smoker recovers from the deepest withdrawal of the entire 24 hour cycle. Human beings naturally wake up feeling relatively refreshed and relaxed after a night's sleep, but the reason a regular smoker soon reaches for a cigarette is not because life presents any stress at this time of day but purely because they are experiencing the worst withdrawal symptoms of the day and need to relieve them.

Is it all beginning to add up? Hopefully the next story will illustrate things even more clearly.

5 - The Rhino

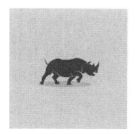

The world is full of drugs that will relax you or give you some kind of lift, but nicotine is not one of those drugs. When you are a smoker you are not just a slave to a drug, you are a slave to a completely useless drug. Throughout this book I've included many of the stories I use in the quit smoking seminars to get this message across more clearly. Sometimes humour and metaphor can communicate the truth better than words, and the more ridiculous the story, the more it is likely to stick in your mind!

Imagine a safari expedition goes wrong. An angry rhino charges a Land Rover terrifying all the tourists inside. Not wanting to kill the animal, the gamekeeper decides to shoot it with tranquillisers. The rhino is shot and falls over on to its side, quickly becoming sedated. It remains there drowsy but unharmed. Further along the track, another rhino appears, also threatening and aggressive. Like the first rhino it charges and almost topples over the Land Rover. However, the gamekeeper has run out of tranquilliser darts and looks around in the back of the vehicle for a fresh supply. He finds none, but comes across a box full of mystery darts. Assuming they are tranquillisers he shoots them into the animal.

At first nothing happens. To everyone's dismay the second rhino does not calm down, instead it appears to become even more worked up. It runs round in circles becoming even more animated and alert. It's metabolism increases, it's body temperature rises and soon everyone realises that the mystery darts contain a stimulant. Luckily, when the rhino charges it misses the vehicle and runs off into the dust until it totally disappears, much to the relief of all concerned.

Everyone knows that a stimulant is the last thing to give a hot blooded animal if you want to calm it down. Stimulants do the opposite to tranquillisers. Knowing this, the passengers turn on the gamekeeper who apologises for his mistake. He tells them about the box of mystery darts and explains that stimulants are only normally used for waking animals up or bringing them out of a coma.

Meanwhile the rhino runs off to the rhino village. He explains to the head rhino, who is also a doctor, that he has been shot. The head rhino examines him, removes the darts, and informs the rhino he has been shot with stimulants. On hearing this the rhino is surprised, saying they didn't make him feel any different to normal. The doctor tells him they are relatively mild and the effect will wear off in a few hours.

Before he lets the patient go the doctor examines one of the darts and notices that although it is a stimulant, it is a well known, quickly addictive drug. He then informs the rhino of this and warns him that although the stimulant effect will quickly wear off, he will then go into withdrawal because he will have already become addicted to the drug.

The rhino is indignant, saying he did not enjoy or even notice the stimulant effect of the drug, and therefore believes he could not possibly go into withdrawal. After all, how can you become hooked on a drug you didn't enjoy?

Actually you can.

And that's exactly what happens when you have your first cigarette. It is a mild stimulant. It does nothing for you, is barely noticeable and everyone assumes they cannot become hooked because they did not enjoy it.

Anyway, back to the story. The rhino goes home to his rhino house. The next day he returns to the doctor. The stimulant effect has long worn off but he is now feeling below par, a little dejected but agitated at the same time. The doctor confirms he is experiencing mild withdrawal but that it will wear off within five or six days. The rhino wanders around the rhino village, pushing young rhinos out of his way, kicking rhino beer cans and feeling miserable. He returns to his rhino job, but finds he irritable. He can't concentrate on his emails or think clearly, he can't relax or enjoy anything. His usual optimism has gone. He wishes there was a way out but the doctor says the only thing he can do is go through the withdrawal. He goes to the rhino pub and has a pint of rhino beer...it's nice... but it does not remove the agitating feeling of withdrawal, in fact if anything, it seems to make it even harder to bear.

A couple of days later he is wandering around the bush, still feeling irritable and empty, still in withdrawal, when the same Land Rover passes by. As it does so a box containing the same stimulant darts falls out of the back of the vehicle and it drives off. The rhino goes up to the box, opens the lid and sees there are 20 darts inside. He realises that if he has another one it will bring him out of withdrawal, so him takes one out and injects it into his hide. The fresh dose relieves all of the withdrawal, he becomes still, he feels a wonderful rush of calm and poses with the dart in his hand, holding it like a cigarette, for all the other animals in the bush to see how cool and relaxed he now is.

He returns to the rhino village and on seeing a group of rhinos, poses with the dart again and says to them:

"Look at me...am I not calm?"

The other rhinos stop what they are doing and agree that they have never before seen such a calm rhino. The rhino doctor comes up and informs the rhino he has re-addicted himself, but the rhino turns to him coolly and says:

"Look at me...am I not the calmest rhino in the whole of Africa?"

The rhino returns to the rhino pub and sits at a table with a pint of rhino beer, holding the stimulant dart aloft in his other hand. Now free of withdrawal, he can enjoy the drink. They seem to go together so well. Other rhinos in the pub look on enviously, wondering what this wonderful new drug must be.

The doctor follows him there and explains that the feeling of elation and satisfaction is not coming from the stimulant, it is only the pleasure of coming out of withdrawal for that drug, reminding him that he did not enjoy it at all the first time, that the drug itself is incapable of doing anything apart from stimulating him, that it cannot providing a feeling of pleasure. The rhino shuts him up, saying how can anyone deny the obvious pleasure he is experiencing?

The doctor informs the rhino that the elation will not last long, that the stimulant will be excreted very soon and then the same withdrawal will return and that each time it will become a little deeper. Over the next few hours the withdrawal indeed returns. The rhino stops feeling confident, he feels deprived, he cannot concentrate on work, he can't relax doing anything. He cannot enjoy rhino TV, he cannot handle stress, all his old feelings of optimism disappear.

So, he returns to the box, there are still 19 stimulants left and so jacks in another one and enjoys the wonderful pleasure all over again. Over the next few days he goes through the process of going down into withdrawal only to take a fresh dart which brings him back to normal. He is now in a circle, a trap. The doctor explains that taking the drug is not a bonus, each stimulant is only capable of bringing him out of withdrawal up to the level of having no withdrawal - the level that all other rhinos are experiencing all day long.

It's exactly the same as smoking. Nicotine is also an addictive stimulant drug that is incapable of relaxing anyone the first time it is taken. Although nobody enjoys the first cigarette, the first dose of nicotine, it then gradually takes you below the level of non smokers into withdrawal. Non smokers never experience withdrawal symptoms. Most smokers believe you have to give up smoking in order to experience them, but the truth is they gradually increase between each cigarette. The smoker then has a choice, He or she can quit smoking and endure the withdrawal symptoms until they eventually disappear over a number of days or weeks...or they can smoke another cigarette, which will relieve the withdrawal but at the same time it will re-addict them. On giving into to the cravings and having another cigarette the smoker relieves those withdrawal symptoms but simply returns to the level that non smokers are experiencing all day long.

After a few days of this dreadful up and down cycle the rhino finally faces the truth. He realises the doctor is right. He has become hooked on a completely useless drug. He takes a spade, digs a deep hole in the ground and celebrates as he buries the remaining stimulants.

It's the same except when you quit smoking there's no need for you to bury anything. Just throw the remaining cigarettes or vapes into the bin, knowing that like the rhino you are giving nothing up, you are freeing yourself from a completely useless drug. If you notice any withdrawal, remember the rhino story. It will remind you that you are escaping from a useless trap and are making no sacrifice whatsoever.

Hopefully, at this point in the book you will already be well on the way to a full understanding as to why nicotine is completely useless and pointless. Before going any further it is useful to look at the dangers of smoking, and how the whole world came to smoke.

Part Two
How Smoking Kills You

"Smoking is the leading cause of statistics" – *Fletcher Knebel*

6 - The Dangers of Smoking

Smoking is a bit like being trapped in a prisoner of war or concentration camp. When planning an escape attempt it's best to get as informed and motivated as possible by finding out what might happen if you choose to remain. So, as your escape navigator, I will outline the risks and "delights" of staying in the camp first, then talk about the escape route - not the other way round. If you are keen to skip ahead do so, but I advise you to return here afterwards and read about the horrors of remaining a smoker. The sequence is not crucial, but if you have the courage to look the dangers in the eye, I advise you to go ahead and read this bit first.

Some authors claim that trying to scare people into stopping smoking is the wrong approach. If it worked, they argue, there'd be hardly anybody left still smoking! After all, most smokers have tried this technique on themselves already, often numerous times...and failed. Some believe that frightening yourself just makes you feel more stressed and maybe even makes you smoke more - and therefore less able to quit. However, in my experience, most smokers are more than happy, or even keen, to look over their shoulder at what they are walking away from, and many are highly motivated to discover how quickly the body repairs itself once they stop.

Almost everybody who decides to quit does so because they are afraid of the consequences of smoking. There's no shortage of horror stories about smoking, but most smokers are unable to make an emotional or intellectual connection with that information because they have become so expert at pushing the fears away as quickly as they can. If you are going to carry on smoking that's maybe the best thing to do. Smoking is stressful enough without having the extra burden of worry, but once you are committed to quitting everything changes. Then, if you have the courage, it's best to turn and face the reality of what smoking or vaping does to your body!

In fact, if you find yourself committed to doing anything in life that is very dangerous, whether it is going up in The Space Shuttle, riding in a motorcycle race, or being in the army, the best thing to do is to put all the risks out of your mind as much as possible, in order to get on and make the most of whatever you are doing. There's no point in constantly worrying about the Space Shuttle crashing, or worry about coming off your bike every time you go round a corner. Constantly thinking of risks isn't a good way to live at all! However, the day you decide to quit forever everything changes. If you really want to stop smoking for good, the best thing to do is to remove the blinkers, and look the dangers and horrors straight in the eye.

7 - Smoking is a bit like being in the army

Actually, being a 20 a day smoker is considerably more dangerous than being in the army, but other than that the two things have a lot in common.

Imagine a doctor in a white coat holding a clipboard visiting an army base in Afghanistan or somewhere. He's been sent to make sure the recruits are informed and warned about the dangers of being in the army. Until his arrival there has been a good atmosphere and lot of laughter coming from the mess and different parts of the base, yet by the time he has spoken to the recruits, they are walking around looking afraid and barely able to concentrate. He goes up to one soldier who is polishing a gun and informs him that he could easily picked off by a sniper, then he speaks to a man about to get into an armoured vehicle and tells him that there's a fairly good chance he could be blown up by a land mine.

The commander hears about the man with the clipboard and tears over towards him asking what the hell he thinks he is doing. The doctor says he is only trying to help, but the commander informs him that his battalion are not stupid and already know the risks. In fact, they had been trying hard to push the risks out of their minds. Most were very good at it, they had surrounded themselves with a protective barrier, a kind of bubble, in which they could forget about the inevitable risks they are taking - bit like a group of smokers chatting and laughing outside a bar. Reminding them about the risks was just making them unhappy and stressed.

There's a lot to be said for this technique of blocking out danger. If you are doing anything truly dangerous, sometimes it's better to harden yourself. The day to dwell on those risks is the day you walk away from them. If you are in the army, the day to think about the reality of the risks is the day you leave, the day you are de-mobbed and are airlifted home. As the helicopter leaves the base you can lower the defensive barrier against the dangers, look down on those poor souls facing their daily next tour of duty and think about what you are getting away from.

The day to face the danger of smoking head on is not when you are sitting outside a bar in the company of other smokers. That's the time to be in denial, to surround yourself with a protective barrier and find comfort in the fact that everyone else seems to be ignoring those risks. The day to face the horrors of smoking is the day you quit. Like the day when a soldier leaves the army.

So assuming you have the courage to take off the protective blinkers and look at the reality of smoking, then read on...

8 - The Stadium

Imagine a vast, empty stadium, perhaps like Wembley Stadium in England. You've arrived there with a young boy you are taking to see a football match, or a big concert. As soon as you get to the car park you realise there are no other cars, nobody else is there, you have obviously got the wrong day. A groundsman sees you standing there, comes up to you, and feeling sorry for the child, opens the gates and allows the two of you to walk onto the pitch.

As you walk across the immaculate, perfectly kept pitch of the deserted stadium the boy forgets his disappointment and is compensated by the walk all the way to the very epicentre of the stadium - the centre circle. He is speechless as he marvels at the enormous sense of space, never having been in a large stadium before. He comments on the greenness of the grass and the blueness of the sky framed above. He is overwhelmed. Then he estimates the number of seats which he guesses to be three or four thousand. You smile and inform him that there are actually 90,000 seats. He cannot begin to comprehend such a large figure and is full of disbelief. He proceeds to count the seats for himself, and being very young, he counts slowly and deliberately, taking ages to reach a hundred. Then, to your relief he gives up at 128. In fact it would take him over a day, literally 25 hours, to count up to 90,000 at the rate of one seat per second.

The silence is broken by a crackle from the loud speaker system and then the two of you hear a clear announcement. To your surprise, you are addressed by name and thanked for coming into the stadium. You are then informed that the true reason you have been invited is to help you stop smoking. Apparently, they are going to fill up the stadium with all the people who died of smoking related illnesses in the United Kingdom over the previous year - so you can see for yourself how many died.

Before they appear, there is a warm up act. Onto the pitch come people who died from using illegal drugs over the last year - class 'A' drugs like heroin, cocaine, ecstasy and LSD. About 247 people slowly make their way onto the pitch representing those who died from Cocaine, followed by 952 people who died from heroin or morphine. You may be surprised to learn that virtually all class 'A' drug victims die from suicide or drug overdose, rather than because of any physical damage caused by the drug. Then 20 people appear who died from taking ecstasy. Nobody was killed that year as a result of taking LSD. After a while, they walk off the pitch leaving it empty again (figures quoted here are from UK Office for National Statistics 2014).

For a minute or two nothing else happens, then there is a drum role, reminiscent of The French Revolution, and as you look towards the players entrance another group of people begin to walk onto the pitch. These are all the people who died over the last twelve months as a result of smoking. Instinctively you study them carefully and to see what they look like, and to your surprise they look very much like a cross section of ordinary looking people, such as you might see in your local shopping centre. Admittedly most of them are middle aged and older, but what you don't like is the occasional younger person coming out. There are beautiful people, plain people, tall people, short people, people of all occupations, healthy, strong looking people and weak looking people alike.

Thousands of them stream onto the pitch. Those who catch your eye almost all look straight at you, as if wanting to tell you something, to warn you not to smoke, but they cannot find the words. What you don't like is the number of young people, some of them in their 20s and 30s, some of them very beautiful. Every single young person you see seems to look down the moment they catch your eye. Just like road accidents and leukemia, smoking is a killer of young people. Dotted around the stadium are young people who died from lung cancer, lip cancer, mouth cancer, throat cancer, and esophageal cancer.

Eventually, several thousand people file out onto the pitch and begin to form a circle around you and the child. They smile at the boy, who smiles back at them, ignorant of the real meaning of their presence. Soon, however, the circle gets smaller and the crowd begin to squash you and the boy together. He become disconcerted and there is inevitable pushing and shoving. Then you begin to feel the crush. The natural dread and fear as the crush worsens is hard to describe. Both you and the boy gasp for breath and then for a whole, terrifying minute you are unable to breath. It feels as if you are someone fighting for their breath in a hospital bed, surrounded by loved ones, possibly fighting the losing battle. A painful battle for breath that can go on for days or weeks, coupled with the knowledge that death is coming.

The boy tumbles down to the ground and holds on to your legs for dear life. You feel his small hands struggling to hold onto you. You imagine how he could not bear to lose you. Down there it is now so dark he can no longer see the green grass or the beautiful, summer sky over head. Then, the crush eases off very slightly as the crowd, having completely filled up the pitch, start to make for the seats. They fill up a hundred seats, then 128, then they fill up a whole block of a thousand. Then two thousand, then 3000, 4000, 5000, 6000, 7000, 8000. Surely there can't be this many people who die every year of smoking related illnesses? After all barely over a thousand died from class A drugs. But the seats keep on filling up, 9000, 10,000, 11,000....When I give my group Quit Smoking Sessions I count all the way up to 90,000.

Incredibly, the number of people who die every year from smoking in The United Kingdom is about 95,000. Some of those who attend the session look shocked as they realise the enormity of annual smoking death, others look a little irritated during the count. Some question the accuracy of the figure. Some are desperate to bury their heads back in the sand and go back to their protective bubble.

Then, everyone in the stadium falls silent, like on Remembrance Day. The sun disappears and the sky becomes overcast. Some people hands and light candles, or ignite lighter flames, as is the custom at large rock concerts. There is the touching and beautiful sight of 95,000 candles, each one representing a life lost to smoking last year. It seems terrible that they all died simply because they smoked. As you comprehend the enormity of the number of people who die every year as a result of smoking you wonder why is it not better known? Why isn't something done about it? How can nature possibly be so cruel to kill all these people every year just because they enjoyed smoking?

Ninety five thousand people every year. That means next year there will be another 95,000 people - and the year after that, and the one after that. It goes on and on. Do they mostly die of lung cancer? Actually, that is a myth. Only about 18,000 people die of lung cancer each year - and that figure includes non smokers. Only about a fifth die of lung cancer, the others die from inflamed lungs, emphysema, blocked arteries, heart attacks, strokes, throat, mouth and esophageal cancer, bladder cancer, plus cancers all over the body. The crowd are then asked to hold up a red card if they were still smoking at the time they were diagnosed with whatever smoking disease killed them. To your surprise, the majority of them hold up a red card. Just by quitting you are drastically cutting down your the chances of death from smoking by 50% - regardless of how long you've smoked or how many you smoke. The body heals itself far more quickly than many health professionals would have you believe. For example, if you quit before the ages of 35-40, the body makes a fairly rapid recovery, and your life expectancy returns to almost the same as someone who has never smoked.

You stand at the epicentre of the enormous stadium, looking over the heads of the 95,000 people. The boy is still desperately holding onto your legs for dear life, terrified of losing you because of smoking. His face is now a grimace of terror. All is now silent, apart from a cough or two in the distance. You realise that every single person is looking at you. You can feel all of them are willing you to stop smoking. Then a solitary voice from about 50 yards away addresses you by name saying:

"Don't smoke ...."

Imagine it is your name being called out. By pure chance you manage to briefly catch the eye of the mystery person despite the distance...their eye seems to twinkle and you realise his or her face is almost identical to your own. Then, a voice quite close behind you in a higher pitched voice also says "Don't smoke" - followed by a succession of others in the enormous crowd start to pick up on your name and you can hear them heckling you from all directions. Some voices are low, some much higher, all kinds of people from all walks of life. It is too late for them but they are all desperate to help you, desperate for you to be aware of the dangers, desperate for you to stop and not share the same fate. You are touched by their concern and eventually you raise your arms as a signal that you are going to make a speech. All falls silent, you pause, then you hear your own voice informing everyone that you are quitting today for many reasons. Each reason gets a ripple of applause. You tell them that you are stopping smoking the moment you finish this book. Thinking of your loved ones, family and friends you tell them solemnly you will never ever smoke another cigarette or take nicotine in any shape or form ever again. The resultant applause is deafening. It sounds louder than Niagara Falls. Most of the crowd now raise their arms up as in salute as they applaud. You can even feel the hands of the little boy down by your legs applauding, his face of terror gone, replaced by a smile of optimism and trust. Does he really understand what is going on? The boy's applause seems to have the greatest effect on you, as if he were your own child, desperate for you to quit and relieved that you are quitting.

Then, as you look around you, you remember that it is too late for all these poor souls in the stadium but you are touched by their support. As the applause dies down you attempt to begin to make your way out of the stadium, but you are hemmed in really tightly and although you push your way through the crowd with strength and determination you seem to move round in circles getting nowhere. Half an hour goes by and you realise you are right back where you started in the centre circle of the pitch. Breaking free from smoking can be tough regardless of your strength and determination.

Then magically the crowd push back and make a narrow pathway through which you can pass. It feels biblical, almost like the Red Sea parting. You and the child make your way along the path towards the exit with people reaching to touch you or pat you on the back as you pass, congratulating you, smiling, cheering you on, some even hugging you. You are touched by the warmth and kindness in their eyes. You are saddened that each one died last year because of smoking. You think of the terror each one of those people must have been through, the grief their deaths must have caused their loved ones and families. You imagine the pain that must still be felt by their children, parents or friends, pain that will go on for many years. Just before you leave the stadium you take one last look at the 95,000. As you do so it is almost nightfall and everyone falls silent again. Many people are taking photographs as they do at a grand opening ceremony or concert. You watch fascinated as countless thousands of the flash and twinkle all over the stadium. Each flash represents a precious life lost to smoking in The United

Kingdom over the last year.

As you watch the spectacle, you ask yourself again how nature can possibly be so cruel as to kill so many people every year just because they enjoyed the comfort and pleasure of smoking? Finally, you make it out of the stadium and find yourself in the main car park, which is sill eerily empty, where you bump into two people. The first is a doctor in a white coat with a clipboard, who wants to lecture you about all the various dangers of smoking. The other, is a native American Indian with an old, wise, swarthy face and a couple of tatty feathers coming from his headdress. Both are keen to speak to you. Instinctively, you choose the Native American Indian.

9 - The Native American Indian

The Native American explains how the people of England came to smoke. Nobody smoked in Europe until 1492 when Columbus and his crew brought tobacco back with them after they discovered America. The Indians had been smoking for thousands of years but Columbus was completely ignorant about smoking. When they were first offered pipes they did not even know whether to suck them or blow them.

Nobody smoked in England until about 1586 - approximately 430 years ago - So there's nothing natural about smoking tobacco. You might think that a cigarette and a drink go naturally together, but whereas alcohol has been around for thousands of years we only started smoking a few centuries ago. That means in 1066 nobody smoked. 1166 nobody smoked. 1266 - minstrels, jousting competitions, playwrights - nobody smoked. Nobody in England had ever seen a pipe. Everyone was completely fine without tobacco, everyone was a non smoker, nobody had any idea what smoking was, till it arrived in The United Kingdom at the end of the Sixteenth century and was popularised by Sir Walter Rayleigh - one of the first ever chain smokers.

It's very patronising to suggest that all the Indians ever smoked was tobacco. History is very vague about why Columbus only came back with tobacco when the Indians smoked so many different things. We now know that the natives were very knowledgeable about drugs, and of course there were no drug laws in those days so they could smoke what they liked. Rather than tobacco, they preferred to smoke other mixtures, such as kirick-kirick, which was made from various plants and tree bark.

They worshiped herbs and plants and knew all about their medicinal properties and narcotic effects. They knew much more than the white man about drugs - they had stimulants the braves could smoke before a battle, and other herbs that could calm you down. They used all kinds of drugs such as salvia and masculine - a hallucinogen which comes from the Peyote Cactus. They did not take any drugs for recreation. Smoking was used exclusively for ceremonies, and for medicinal purposes - it was a central part of their culture. Blowing smoke into the air was a way they communicated with the Gods.

Crucially, they didn't inhale the smoke. The practice of inhaling tobacco smoke into the lungs was introduced by the white man. The Indians warned us that tobacco could bring death if used inappropriately, but sadly, they were ignored.

The natural, traditional strains of tobacco the Indians smoked were much darker, rougher and bitter tasting - think of a very coarse cigar smoke and you will soon understand why the smoke was never inhaled. They just sucked the smoke into their mouths and blew it out, as if blowing smoke signals to the Gods, it was not being used for recreation. Although tobacco was looked upon as a sacred plant, the Indians never appeared to become hooked or dependent upon nicotine - they were the equivalent of the modern day occasional smoker, rather than the typical all day long habit of the modern era. They rarely smoked recreationally, nor become addicted as the sailors and settlers quickly did. They didn't have to get out of the tepee every morning and smoke a pipe before they could face the day like the typical modern day smoker! Some tribes chewed tobacco for recreational use and this practice was also adopted by the settlers.

It is quite possible that the Indians kept the more important ingredients of their pipes a secret from the white man, which would explain why Columbus came back only with tobacco - but it is unlikely we will ever know the truth. However, it would not be surprising because the recipes of the pipes were sacred to them. The elders would typically not even share the ingredients with younger members of the tribes and would certainly not share them with other tribes.

There are over 60 species of tobacco growing wild in most sections of North America. However, the original, real tobacco is in no way related to modern commercially grown strains - which are specially cultivated to be much milder, and have a much higher nicotine content. Once the practice of inhaling the smoke into the lungs began the sailors very easily became hooked. The quickly addictive nature of nicotine meant it spread rapidly over mainland Europe. The lighter strains of tobacco favoured by the Spanish were problematic and would not stay alight, so potassium nitrate was added as an incendiary - the same substance used in gunpowder and sparklers. It is still an ingredient in modern cigarettes. When smoked alone tobacco does not stay alight in the natural world, but the Indians did not encounter this problem as they rarely, if ever, smoked tobacco alone.

Basically, it was all a terrible mistake. To summarise - the people who gave us tobacco smoked much more natural strains, they didn't inhale the fumes, and normally smoked it as a mixture with other herbs and drugs. Their warning that tobacco could bring death was ignored and forgotten through the ignorance, or possibly even arrogance of the settlers from Europe.

Some historians make out the native tribes of the Caribbean Islands habitually smoked primitive cigars recreationally. According to the sailor's logs in 1492 the natives wafted aromatic smoke from what looked like massive, trumpet shaped objects in front of the new arrivals - but this display could easily have been in honour of the sailors because the arrival of their ships was a *special event*, not a display of recreational smoking. Remember, smoking was a way they communicated with their Gods and asked for protection. Creating smoke with various fragrances was a crucial and frequent part of all their ceremonies, rather like in Roman Catholic ceremonies, smoke is wafted all over the place in the form of incense!

10 - The Spread of Smoking

The white man's habit of smoking recreationally spread very quickly - by the mid 1500s it was spreading north from Spain into France and tobacco was soon being cultivated all over Europe. Tobacco leaves have to be dried before they can be smoked, but the Spanish had trouble curing the tobacco and keeping it fresh, lacking the knowledge of the Indians. It was easier simply to chew it, so chewing tobacco and snuff (sniffing the ground leaves up the nose) remained more popular than smoking until the mid 1800s. The addiction of potassium nitrate began a process removing tobacco smoking further and further away from nature. Other poisonous incendiaries, along with countess chemical additives and artificial flavourings are now packed into modern cigarettes.

Right up till the mid 1880s, taking snuff was far more popular than smoking. Women did not smoke at all, preferring snuff, which, like all forms of tobacco was considered to be medicinal. By the time of the Great Plague in 1666 snuff became popular in elite circles, when even royal women carried around special boxes. Cigarettes (French for "little cigar") first appeared in Seville in the mid 1700s but did not become fashionable until the Crimean War in the mid Nineteenth Century. By now smoking had overtaken snuff taking, and in 1880, after the invention of the first cigarette making machines, pipes were gradually replaced by cigarettes.

Previous to The First World War hardly any women smoked. Nurses on the front line were handed cigarettes by men, but until the 1930s only a tiny percentage of women smoked. Today almost as many women smoke as men, and the number one cause of female death is now Lung Cancer, which was previously very rare. Few women realise that the sole reason they began to smoke en masse was because they were specifically targeted by an ingenious advertising campaign in 1929. The man behind it was Edward Bernays. He bribed female movie stars to smoke in their movies, and encouraged women to think that smoking symbolised liberation from male domination. His "Torches of Freedom" ad campaign made out that smoking gave women independence, sophistication, glamour, and sexual allure. Rather than finding freedom they were sold an addiction. The tobacco companies knew that if they could persuade women to smoke they would double their sales. It worked - the campaign was so successful that within just a few years they achieved their goal

11 - Modern Cigarettes

Ammonia, sugars, saccharin are now added in cigarette factories so that the nicotine absorption rate is higher - making cigarettes more addictive. The effect of ammonia alone is quite considerable. Other chemicals are added to make the smoke smoother and silkier - remember in the natural state tobacco smoke is very rough and more like inhaling a bonfire. Artificial flavourings are added, such as Diacetyl - a chemical which is known to cause irreversible scaring of the lungs.

Filters are made from cellulose acetate. Interestingly, the first filter tips - on Kent Cigarettes - were made of asbestos. Filters and low tar cigarettes followed the lung cancer scare of the 1960s and actually boosted sales because they were a clever ploy to reassure people. They actually make no difference whatsoever to the incidence of lung disease.

Radiation

When you smoke modern cigarettes you are also breathing in dangerous amounts of a radioactive substances such as polnium-210, which can accumulate and form radioactive clusters or "hot spots" in the lungs. This acts like a time bomb in terms of bronchial cancer risk (Radford and Hunt 1964).

Tobacco companies have tried in vain to create a radiation free cigarette using special washing techniques and filters, but all attempts so far have failed. Tobacco contains radiation naturally, because the leaves are covered in sticky hairs, making them especially good at catching chemicals from the atmosphere around them, including radioactive elements. Since the 1950s many tobacco plants are grown using phosphate fertilisers that contain a mineral known as apatite. Apatite contains radium, which can eventually decay into polonium-210.

People sometimes wonder how nature can be so cruel as to cull stadium loads of people each year as a result of smoking tobacco, but in fact, nature isn't cruel at all. After a five hundred year experiment with smoking, it's pretty clear that we simply aren't supposed to inhale tobacco, we weren't supposed to add chemicals and certainly should not smoke it all day long. The people who gave us tobacco certainly didn't do any of these things. It seems they chewed tobacco for recreational use rather than using it for smoking, but they discovered one other use for tobacco...

...they used it as an insecticide.

12 - Nicotine is an insecticide

The Native Americans were ingenious and knowledgeable, they knew all about poisonous plants like tobacco and were one of the first peoples of the world to use insecticides. They were so ahead of their time that the civilised world did not start using insecticides until the Twentieth Century.

The tobacco plant is very clever. Most insects and pests won't eat it because the poison in the leaves kills them. Humans can therefore use this to their advantage, by using this poison as an insecticide. It's a cheap way of making an insecticide and a very powerful one too because nicotine is neurotoxic to many insects. Spray in on the crops and the insects shrivel up and die. It's the most deadly natural insecticide in the world and is on a par with many pharmaceutical insecticides, such as Imidacloprid (the world's most widely used insecticide) which is actually a synthetic form of nicotine. Nicotine is banned in many countries but still used all over the third world because it is a cheap and effective.

Gardeners in England used to keep the ash from their ashtrays, add water and use it as an insecticide paste! Imagine being given an insecticide by a farmer and being told to inhale it 20 times a day! Who on earth in their right mind would do that to their body?...But If you are a smoker who gets through a packet a day, there's no need - you already do this.

Nicotine isn't just a drug, it is one of the most poisonous natural substances on the planet. It's more deadly ounce for ounce than arsenic or strychnine. It is also a neurotoxic to humans if not excreted rapidly from the body. In fact, the nicotine from one cigar would kill a human being were it to be injected into a vein. Even one drop of pure nicotine on the back of the hand would be enough to kill. The lethal dose 40 to 60 mg and every cigarette contains between 4-14 mg.

The deadly nature of nicotine wasn't fully appreciated by the scientific or medical community until well into the Twentieth Century, when the Scottish doctor Lennox Johnston published his book *The Disease of Tobacco Smoking and Its Cure* (1957). He began to experiment with nicotine injections. By accident, he sprayed just a few drops of 40% nicotine solution on to his hand, to his complete surprise and horror, he collapsed and almost died. Nicotine patches can even be lethal if the skin beneath them splits. This should give you an idea why vaping, which is basically inhaling pure nicotine, can be as harmful as smoking.

Nicotine appears to act as a pathway for cancer in various ways. Rather than initiating cancer, it seems create an environment that promotes cancer development and growth and can make existing cancers more aggressive (Sanner and Grimsrud 2015). Evidence is also emerging of direct contributions of nicotine to cancer onset and growth. The list of cancers reportedly connected to nicotine is expanding and presently includes small-cell and non-small-cell lung carcinomas, as well as head and neck, gastric, pancreatic, gallbladder, liver, colon, breast, cervical, urinary bladder and kidney cancers (Grando 2014).

Many smokers begin to feel a little below par as they stub out a cigarette. Drug levels are actually at their highest at this point but the body has just received a big dose of poison. During and after each cigarette the body has to excrete nicotine as quickly as possible to prevent serious damage to the brain and it does this very efficiently - but at a cost. The reason a typical smoker feels tired and lethargic so often isn't because their lungs are full of tobacco tar (which they are) but because of the energy needed to constantly excrete the poison of nicotine all day long. Smokers are literally being poisoned. All cigarette smoke carries a deadly cargo of nicotine. This is most likely the main reason first time smokers experience nausea and other unpleasant reactions. It's not just a reaction, it's also the body's natural way of warning us as to the presence of a new poison.

if you inhale cigarette smoke or nicotine vapour you do not die, because you are not an insect, however, many cells in the mouth and periodontal ligaments are irritated and killed by the nicotine. This is because nicotine doesn't differentiate between insect cells and the ones in the human body. Nicotine kills cells in the lungs which then drop down, mix with bacteria and form smokers phlegm, explaining why smoker's phlegm is just as common in people who choose to vape rather than smoke. In fact vaping often causes more phlegm than smoking because the vapour is more or less pure nicotine, in other words, pure insecticide.

People who smoke or vape with the same part of the mouth or lips sometimes notice discolouration, ulcers or rough skin developing. This is a warning sign. Smoking related cancer sometimes starts with a lump or sore patch in the mouth or on the lips which won't go away.

Saliva clears away much of the deadly nicotine and other poisons from the mouth in between cigarettes, or vapes, otherwise mouth cancer would be far more common, but once swallowed...it makes its way down the esophagus. Some people are puzzled as to why esophageal cancer is a smoking related illness at all, and wonder why it is so much more common amongst smokers compared to non smokers, but is it really any surprise when you consider that cigarettes provide a slow delivery of an insecticide into the esophagus all day long? Esophageal tissues are quite fragile. Obviously all of the smoke goes into the lungs, but tobacco tar is only one of the many dangers of smoking.

Cigar and pipe smokers may not usually inhale so much smoke but just like cigarette smokers, they have a much increased incidence of esophageal and stomach cancer, many times that of non smokers.

If you have ever broken open the filter tip of a cigarette and compared the appearance before and after smoking you will have seen how badly tobacco tar stains. Each cigarette is staining the precious membranes of your lungs in the same way, and as it accumulates, it forms a sticky, dark residue. Tobacco tar is the world's most aggressive, natural carcinogen and if you are a smoker it is in your lungs right now! If you smoke 20 cigarettes a day, roughly a coffee cup of that tar forms in the lungs every year. Lung material is light and spongy, a bit like a kitchen or bathroom sponge. Imagine going into your kitchen and finding that someone had used your best sponge to mop up filthy, dark brown sticky stuff from the floor! You'd be horrified. You'd probably want to throw that sponge away - probably the best idea - but when it's your own lungs, then what? You can't just throw them away and get a new pair. The colour of the tar in a smoker's lungs has to be seen to be believed, and the stickiness is disgusting! A non smokers lungs are a bright pinky, healthy colour, but those of a smoker are very dark brown - often black in places. Luckily the body is like a very efficient washing machine, and when you quit the majority of tar is removed from the lungs in the first year of being a non smoker, plus of course, no new tar is formed. The lungs return pretty much to normal in approximately seven years. The manufacturers of Marlborough cigarettes famously ran an advertising campaign running for nearly 50 years using a character known as The Marlborough Cowboy, in an attempt to give filter tipped cigarettes a rugged, masculine image. This was because tipped cigarettes were previously associated with women smokers. It worked, men became happy to smoke cigarettes with filter tips and sales increased by billions of dollars. In the end, it backfired, the actor who played The Marlborough Cowboy died of lung cancer, so did another actor who replaced him. In total six men who played the role died from lung illness caused by smoking.

Light and intermittent smoking is almost as dangerous as heavy smoking, especially with regard to lung cancer and heart disease (Rebecca Schane 2010). Light and intermittent smokers often do not view themselves as smokers, but on average, every 15th cigarette smoked causes the DNA of a healthy cell somewhere in the body to mutate. DNA damage from smoking is thought to be irreversible, so even an occasional cigarette can one day bring about cancer of the lip, tongue, mouth, throat, esophagus, lungs or anywhere in the body. The best thing to do is to stop now!

When I first carried out quit smoking groups in the late 1990s I used to show pictures of mouth, tongue, laryngeal and throat cancer to all the participants. On the wall of the office was a well known picture of a woman suffering from throat cancer who could now only breath through a special hole beneath her larynx. Despite her condition she was still addicted to cigarettes and is shown smoking a cigarette through this breathing hole in her neck. Before she died, she wanted the picture circulated to as many people as possible in the hope it would show how addictive smoking is, and deter other people from starting.

We also made a video of a doctor in Charring Cross Hospital explaining how people with smoking related illness often die in terrible distress or pain, sometimes fighting to breathe for days on end because of smoking related cancers, and how, for example, healthy teeth need to be extracted before radiotherapy treatment can be carried out to treat some forms of mouth cancer.

There is a widespread myth that most smoking related deaths are caused by lung cancer. This myth is often supported by the media and organisations who focus almost entirely on the risk of lung cancer when encouraging people to stop smoking. Lung cancer may be the greatest risk to smokers but it only accounts for approximately one fifth of all smoking related deaths, in UK it causes roughly 18,000 out of the total of 95,000 or so smoking related deaths each year. As many smokers die from other lung diseases, such as emphysema and chronic bronchitis as die from lung cancer. Throat cancer and heart disease and other big risks.

Many people are puzzled as to why smoking leads to heart disease, after all, the tobacco tar remains within the lungs. When I do group quit smoking sessions, I sometimes ask if anybody knows why smoking is linked to heart disease or blocked arteries. Usually no one has the slightest idea. The tar goes no further than the lungs but nicotine is transported all over the body by the blood stream and remember, it is an insecticide. Nicotine is a vasoconstrictor, which means it narrows the blood vessels all over the body, including the coronary arteries that feed the heart muscle. In addition, smoking causes arteries throughout the body to become lined with fatty deposits. If you look at a cross section taken from the artery of a smoker, you can see fatty deposits that are reminiscent of water pipes being furred up with lime scale. Not surprisingly, smokers are far more likely to die of a stroke, due to the narrowing of blood vessels in the brain.

Smoking effects sexual performance in men, and impotence is far more common in men who smoke because the blood supply to the penis is gradually reduced by the same process. Recent studies have found that smoking reduces sperm count in men by about 23%, decreases the ability of sperm to swim and deviates how sperm are shaped (Michael OlekJ 2016; Sharma et al 2016).

Every year, thousands of smokers have their legs amputated because of peripheral arterial diseases like Buergers disease. This occurs when the blood supply to the legs or arms is seriously impaired by damage to the vascular system. Buergers disease is unknown amongst non smokers. I read a newspaper article recently about a woman from Liskeard, Cornwall, Victoria Marks, who gave up smoking when she was 31, but 10 years after she quit she was diagnosed with Buerger's disease and had to have both legs amputated. She wanted her story broadcast as widely as possible to avert others to the danger of this disease, so I have given her a mention here. Victoria believes more should be done to tell others about the lesser known dangers of smoking.

Although scientists know that smoking leads to higher cancer rates for almost every part of the human body, they do not fully understand the mechanisms involved. However, we do know that fighting off cancer at the very earliest stage depends on the integrity of the body's immune system. Having such a high level of poison in the body the whole time depletes antioxidants and therefore compromises the immune system. We also know that any cigarette can cause mutations in DNA, mutated cells or deviant cells. If these cells are not identified and destroyed by the immune system it can lead to cancer almost anywhere in the body. These deviant cells are forming every time you smoke, even if you are a light smoker or just an occasional smoker. The only way to stop this happening is to stop smoking completely.

13 - If a pregnant woman smokes - baby smokes too

Everybody knows that it is especially inadvisable for pregnant women to smoke. The tobacco tar remains in the lungs, so obviously it doesn't reach the growing baby, but nicotine does. Nicotine is a vasoconstrictor which narrows the arteries throughout the body, including those supplying oxygen to the baby, and remember, it is an insecticide. Smoking causes a chronic elevation in carbon dioxide levels, meaning the growing baby is starved of the normal amount of oxygen. Not surprisingly, this can effect organ development, the baby's growth is always restricted if the mother smokes, and complications during pregnancy, such as ectopic pregnancy (pregnancy in the fallopian tube) are far more common. Smoking during pregnancy is linked to cot deaths, infant mortality, and birth defects such as cleft palette and missing eyes - reminiscent of the deformities that can result from inhaling insecticides.

Even snuff is known to be damaging to newborn babies. A study by Michael Seigel (2011) showed how nicotine in snuff may disrupt the development of a newborn's nervous system, causing breathing problems.

Would you advise a pregnant woman to work in a farm where insecticide is sprayed several times a day? Of course not, most people would agree there was a risk of causing abnormalities to the unborn child. If a woman smokes say, twenty cigarettes a day, then there is no need for her to work on that farm. She is delivering twenty doses of an insecticide directly to her baby in any case.

Pregnancy aside, every organ in the body is subjected to nicotine if you smoke or vape. Hardly surprising then that smoking is the number one cause of, for example, bladder cancer. Women who smoke also face an increased risk of breast cancer and gynecological cancers, particularly cervical cancer, which has a very strong association.

Recent research suggests that all cancer is caused by mutations in the DNA of a cell. A study by Ludmil Alexandrov et al (2016) analyzed over 5,000 tumors, comparing cancers from smokers with those from people who had never smoked. The results showed that a smoking a packet of cigarettes a day led to an average 150 mutations within every single cell in the lungs, 97 mutations in each cell in the larynx, 39 mutations for the pharynx, 23 for the mouth, 18 for the bladder, and six mutations in every cell of the liver each year.

14 - Smoking ages you

N othing ages you like smoking. Women smokers in particular are well aware of the fact that smoking gives you wrinkles as you get older, but they are not usually so aware of the fact that every single cigarette ages them.

It's not really so surprising when you recall that nicotine is an insecticide, and every cigarette is delivering that insecticide and many other poisons to your skin. Almost as soon as you start smoking you begin to lose that very special bloom of youthful vitality. Every cigarette is chasing it further away. You look younger for longer if you never smoke. Looking older and more mature may appeal to young teenage boys but rarely to women. Middle aged women who smoke often look considerably older than their years because of the tell tale wrinkles around the mouth, that look like stitch marks. They get terrible wrinkles, dark areas and puffiness around the eyes caused by smoking, plus sometimes a sallow or orange appearance to the skin. Even if you are a light smoker you are damaging the skin with each cigarette. Each cigarette depletes vitamin C levels by about 25mg - that's about the same amount you get in a typical orange. Vitamin C is an essential antioxidant that removes poisons from the body and keeps skin young looking and elastic. Nicotine also reduces vitamin E levels which is also vital for the skin. A woman may be using the most expensive creams and lotions available in the world in an attempt to look younger, but if she is smoking, she is losing the battle from the inside.

The aging cream

If there was a cream you could buy from the chemist that was guaranteed to age you, just a little bit, every time you put it on your face (and the effects were permanent) nobody would buy it. When you are smoker there is no need to buy that cream - because every cigarette is doing the job for you, it is aging you anyway! This applies whether you are a heavy smoker, light smoker or even an occasional smoker. The more you smoke, the more damage you are doing to your skin. The damage to the exterior is visible, whereas damage to internal organs is invisible. The skin gives you an indication of what you are doing to the inside your body.

Fatter waist

A very large study looking at smoking habits of over 147,000 people showed that smoking causes an increase in fat stored around the waist. The more cigarettes smoked the greater the effect (Richard Morris et al 2015).

Remember, there is nothing natural about habitually inhaling tobacco. The people who gave us tobacco, the Native American Indians, rarely inhaled the smoke. They warned us that smoking could bring death. I make no apology for bombarding you with all this information about the dangers of smoking. Nothing is exaggerated, there is no need for exaggeration because the horrors of smoking are bad enough. I've focused on fatal illnesses that smoking can give you but there are almost as many non fatal illnesses such as angina, high blood pressure and a form of blindness known as macular degeneration.

What it all adds up to is there is a strong likelihood that smoking, at some stage, will kill you. By now, you should be in absolutely no doubt that smoking is a useless trap, and maybe even looking forward to your escape, but there are still a number of useful things for you to know that will help you on your way to quitting with the minimum of trauma.

Blood pressure

You may not notice the very slight stimulant action of nicotine when you smoke or vape, but each dose raises your blood pressure for approximately four hours. This is because nicotine constricts blood vessels all over the body. This means that once you become a smoker it's not so easy to relax as it was before you started smoking. It's harder to sleep, harder to handle stress, harder to handle difficult situations. If you get into a disagreement with someone, your blood pressure is already too high, so it's even harder to stay cool.

Nicotine also contributes to insulin resistance an increased risk for type 2 diabetes, especially in overweight smokers.

Smokers feel tired and lethargic

Nothing saps your energy, power, stamina and strength like smoking, which is why professional sport people never smoke. Physically you are way below your full potential if you smoke because the removal of nicotine and other poisons is a perpetual strain on the body.

Apart from killing you, smoking makes you constantly feel tired and lethargic. If you smoke every day you will likely feel jaded and below par much of the time without maybe realising it is because of smoking. This is not because of the buildup of tar in the lungs but because of the body's constant need to divert energy and resources into removing the toxins of smoking. Nicotine must be removed from the body as soon as possible after smoking. If allowed to accumulate it would destroy brain cells and therefore the body diverts and depletes resources in order to excrete the drug. It's a bit like having a very mild illness every day of your life, such as a low grade cold or infection. The reason most bacteria or viruses cause us to feel ill is not their actual presence, it is due to the toxins they excrete. Stopping smoking isn't just another detox, it is the detox of your life.

Smoking takes the edge of our sparkle and vitality because of the energy the body diverts in order to excrete nicotine and other poisons. You would likely feel the same way if you consumed small quantities of a poison like arsenic at regular intervals every day. Remember, ounce per ounce, nicotine is more deadly than arsenic. Feeling slightly run down in this way makes it even more difficult to endure the withdrawal symptoms for nicotine, which gradually increase between each cigarette, and light up again, thus perpetuating the trap.

15 - Russian Roulette

Smoking kills about one in four smokers before the end of middle age. That means, statistically speaking, smoking is more dangerous than fighting in World War One! (Nine million lost their lives out of a total of 65,000 military personnel, which is about one in seven).

Imagine playing Russian Roulette in front of a group of children, possibly your own. First you ask them to stop playing with their toys and turn round to look round at you. Then as soon as they fall silent, you lift up a real hand gun and tell the children you are going to play a game. You are going to pull the trigger in a few seconds time. Their smiles fade and are replaced by looks of terror. You inform the children that the odds are one in six that you will survive...there are six chambers in the gun and only one will contain a bullet. You place the bullet in the gun and spin round the chambers, then you hold the gun to the side of your head. You notice the feeling of the cold metal on your head and become aware of the surprising heaviness of the gun.

Before pulling the trigger, you pause to look at the children's faces. One begins to cry, another trembles, a third throws up, but you ignore all this.

The chances are 6-1 that you would survive....but would you ever really do this?

Well, you don't need to go to all that bother if you remain being a smoker, because you are taking an even greater risk with your life. One in four smokers will die before or during middle age. Some surveys put the figure at one in three. That would mean you'd have to put would have to put two bullets in the gun, or play Russian Roulette twice!

16 - You never reach your full potential

The sad fact is, if you continue smoking there will never be a day in your life when reach your full potential as a man or a woman. Not in terms of looks, muscle strength, fitness, stamina, health, or sexual performance. Your hair and clothes will smell like a smokey dustbin every time you smoke, your mouth will taste like an ashtray and your teeth will constantly be discoloured.

Cigarettes do not just kill a specific group of people. It's no joke dying fighting for your breath, or from cancer of the lip caused by smoking. It can happen to any smoker. We always think it's on the other side of the fence but no one is immune to the dangers of tobacco, not the young, the strong and healthy, not celebrities, not light smokers or occasional smokers. Even non-smokers exposed to secondhand smoke are at risk.

Does the drug make it all worth it? The biggest irony of all is that nicotine is not only useless, it makes you more stressed and less able to relax in every situation in life.

The next part of the book is a further, more detailed look at why nicotine is useless. That message has been broken into two waves, with the dangers of smoking coming in the middle, in order that the initial message has a chance to sink in, and to avoid information overkill. This is because the idea that smoking is pointless from a drug perspective goes against the grain of everything most of us have believed all of our lives.

Part Three
Why Nicotine is Useless
(cont.)

17 - The Nicotine Delusion - Part Two

Hopefully, when you read Part One of The Nicotine Delusion something already clicked or shifted within you. With any luck you began to understand why every single cigarette you ever smoked was pointless.

When I carry out quit smoking sessions, even during the latter stages you still get people who just can't come to terms with why nicotine is constantly being referred to as a *useless* drug. The assumption that nicotine has obvious benefit is deeply ingrained into the psyche of almost everyone, so when they are first introduced to the notion that it has no benefit whatsoever they can't truly accept it. After all, why haven't they heard this from scientists and doctors? Why haven't they heard this message from the media or from quit smoking organisations? Either the message does not truly convince them or they still just can't quite understand it. Here's the message in a nutshell again:

"It is not the drug nicotine itself that brings about any pleasure - one hundred percent of the pleasure from smoking or vaping comes from relieving the withdrawal symptoms that crop up between each cigarette or dose."

I realise it can be difficult to accept - after all when someone smokes or vapes there's an undeniable lift, a hit, a rush, a feeling of elation or satisfaction... call it what you like. Smokers know the harm they are doing to themselves, they want to be free, but they just can't get to grips with the notion that nicotine is useless and that by quitting they are making no sacrifice. Some are still nervous about life as a non smoker and ask me questions like:

How will I relax without cigarettes? How will I cope with stress? How will I be able to concentrate? How will I think things through deeply? How will I handle not having a reward when I've completed things? How will I get going? How will I handle rows? What will I do after food? How will I get "me" time? What will I look forward to?

They are correct in that smoking or vaping can provide help or pleasure in all of those situations but that is not why the drug nicotine is useless. Rather than repeating why nicotine is useless over and over again, sometimes it's much more powerful and entertaining to illustrate what is being said by using comparisons or metaphors until everything really sinks in.

As a hypnotist with many years working at the sharp end with smokers, I am aware of the power of mental imagery. It's often used in a technique known as Neuro Linguistic Programming (NLP) plus it's a lot more memorable.

Everything you need to know about why smoking or vaping is useless is contained in each of these crazy stories. I once read that if you are creating an analogy, the crazier and wackier ones are most likely to drive home the point and be remembered the longest. It is an especially useful way of remembering why nicotine is a pointless drug. So here is the next NLP metaphor - the Strappie Story.

18 - The Strappie Story

As you return to daily life as a non smoker you will come across situations and times when, typically you used to smoke. The following story will help you recall why nicotine is useless, and even amuse you when you encounter those situations.

Imagine you're visiting a very strange country where people tend to sit outside cafés and bars in the evenings, wearing very tight straps around their forearms, that look a bit like the kind of things a punk or heavy metal singer might wear - very tight, thick, large straps around their entire forearms. Men and women are all wearing them and you're curious to know why.

As you sit in one of the cafés you notice that most of the strap wearers appear to be a little subdued. One man in particular glances every now and then down at his strap. You ask him why he is wearing such a large, tight thing around his wrist and he explains to you that once you get used to them they can give you a wonderful feeling of pleasure. It is now almost an hour since he put his strap on. He tells you it was very comfortable back then, he felt relaxed and could handle his day easily. He could handle work and leisure, but as time has gone by the strap has slowly got tighter. At first he didn't really notice the tightness and could ignore the strap but it's now been on a whole hour and is affecting his mood. He is desperate to remove it. He is becoming restless.

At that moment a timer attached to the strap bleeps, indicating that it has now been on a whole hour. With great pleasure the man presses the release button and the whole strap falls off. Suddenly he is completely relaxed, his mood lifted. He looks relieved and satisfied. He then holds the strap aloft with his other hand looking around him with a calm and serene expression on his face. His whole mood seems to transform. He now seems at ease and happier, his body language more confident. He looks around at everyone in the bar with a look of self assurance, then at me, asking if I now understand the reason for wearing the strap. Apparently, it is to obtain the incredible pleasure I am now witnessing. He then gazes into the distance, still posing with the strap aloft in one hand, looking as calm and in control as Clint Eastward.

His elation lasts for a minute or two but then gradually evapourates, the reason for which is obvious. The whole pleasure he just experienced was simply that of returning to normal, returning to how he felt before he put the thing on. The pleasure was simply relief at escaping from the increasing tension the strap had been causing him. Now back to normal all the tension had left both his mind and body. You had never seen a calmer man.

To your amazement, he proceeds to put the strap back on, telling you it will feel completely comfortable at first but that it is fitted with a device to make it gradually get tighter over the next hour. He replaces the strap and initially it is comfortable and unnoticeable. There is a controller on the strap that sets the rate at which it gets tighter. It is currently set for one hour but you can set it so that the strap doesn't reach full tightness for several hours or even days.

Apparently at times when he is busy he doesn't notice the strap at all, even when it steadily becomes tighter, but as it gradually worsens he becomes only too aware of the increasing tightness and looks forward to removing it when the hour is up. Usually his mood begins to decline as the tightness increases, a bit like going down a flight of steps. The further down the steps of tightness he goes, the worse his mood becomes.

Another hour goes by, during which his relaxed mood gradually fades and is replaced by tension. At the end of the hour the strap bleeps, he presses the release, and it falls off again. Once again his mood abruptly changes and he enjoys the feeling of complete serenity and calm again.

Sometimes, instead of waiting for the whole hour to be up, he can't resist pressing the release button early, say for example when there is a period of stress or boredom. He finds that removing the strap strategically at these times aids concentration, allows him to think more clearly and gives him a little lift that non strap wearers do not get.

You look around at some of the other strap wearers in the café. Those whose straps are at the tight stage are looking a bit fed up or miserable compared to the non strap wearers. Some strap wearers look subdued whereas others look irritable and restless. Suddenly there is a bleep from the strap being worn by a very attractive woman quite close to you. She looks relieved and smiles with anticipation, even before she presses the release button. Her strap falls off and she instantly looks calmer. She lifts her strap aloft, posing with it confidently in one hand. She looks around the bar now beaming, looking serene and confident now the strap is off. She catches your eye and smiles as if to say:

"Look at me. Look how elegant and sophisticated I am holding my tight strap aloft in my hand"

You speak to her and comment on how relaxed and in control she now appears to be. She nods knowingly in agreement. Apparently she is only a light strap user. She sets the timer on her strap to go off once a week. This means it gets tighter much more slowly and remains comfortable for a much longer period, but gradually the tightness increases until by the time the week is up she is looking to removing it and can think of little else.

Then someone else's strap timer bleeps. You turn to this person. You'd noticed him earlier, as being probably the most miserable and edgy looking man in the entire café, but as soon as his strap is released he begins to laugh easily and spontaneously at the slightest thing. His mood has clearly been completely transformed by removing the strap. Seeing how impressed you are at the obvious benefit the strap wearers are enjoying, the woman advises you to buy one for yourself so that you can share the pleasure. Apparently they are affectionately known as "strappies". Anyone over 16 can purchase them. So you take one back home with you to try out after the holiday.

The strappie is surprisingly comfortable when you first put it on, and you set the tightness timer at the lowest setting, so that it does not become tight for three days. You forget you are wearing it for the first couple of days and even when sleeping at night it is unnoticeable. At the beginning of the third day the tightness begins to get to you and consequently it affects your mood. You are less relaxed than usual and very much looking forward to removing the strap. That evening when you are sitting outside a bar the timer goes off and the feeling of elation when you press the release is overwhelming. You feel so relieved and happy. It is by far the best moment of the entire day. Your mood lifts sky high and you feel much more relaxed and sociable. A few minutes later your forearm returns to normal and the feeling subsides. You then replace the strappie on its lowest setting and forget it until the next three days are almost up when once again the bleep sounds, you remove the strap. Immediately you get the same wonderful lift again. You feel relaxed, serene and calm. The nagging desire to remove the strap has gone.

After this you decide to change the strappie timer. You increase the tightness rate so that it reaches full tightness every day. This means you now get to enjoy the same amazing feeling every single day! So for the next week you press the release once a day just after you have returned home from work. You start to really look forward to the strap coming off after work.

You are tempted to gradually increase the timer so that the strap gets tighter at even shorter intervals, meaning you will get the pleasure of removing it even more often. Eventually you set it so that it is going off twenty times a day - meaning you now have twenty wonderful moments to look forward to every single day. You are now a confirmed stappie wearer.

Amazingly the strappie is unnoticeable when you are asleep, but soon after waking up you are keen to remove it. You also enjoy removing it while you have your morning tea or coffee. You then replace it and set off to work but half way to work it is already uncomfortable again and so you have to remove it just before you go into the office. You are fine wearing the strap for the first hour or so of work but after that you can barely concentrate. Every time the strap comes off your concentration seems to be perfect. You enjoy nipping outside for a strappie break several times a day.

Witnessing the obvious pleasure the strappie gives you, several friends and work colleagues buy one for themselves. Soon you are enjoying strappie breaks together. One of your colleagues removes her strappie just before going into meetings, so that the meeting isn't spoilt by the desire to remove the strap, and she can think more clearly. By the end of each meeting however she finds it has become tight again, so the first thing he does afterwards is enjoy removing it.

In the evenings she generally removes the strap four or five times, unless she is drinking alcohol, in which case she ends to take it off far more often. Her willpower to leave the strap on for more than a few minutes seems to diminish once she's had a few drinks. Consequently she does not leave it on long enough to get sufficiently tight - and therefore gets progressively less pleasure when she takes it off.

A male colleague finds it is useful to remove his strappie whenever he has a row with his girlfriend. Half way through one row he notices he has two sets off stress. Half the stress is his irritation with his unreasonable girlfriend, and the other half is the tension from the strappie which he has not removed for almost an hour. So he goes out into the garden, removes the strap and consequently halves his stress! With half of his stress now gone he returns back inside and finds it so much easier to handle his girlfriend.

A few weeks later you finally realise that strappie wearing, though offering a huge pleasure every time the strap is removed, is a complete waste of time. It is utterly pointless. Most of your friends and colleagues have come to the same conclusion, and ceremoniously, you all cast your strappies into a bin and forget about them.

It all goes well...but the colleague with the difficult girlfriend finds it hard being an ex-strappie wearer. He keeps casting his mind back to the lovely feeling he enjoyed whenever he took his strappieoff. He even misses the familiar feeling of pressing the release button. He has golden memoriesof how strappies used to help him concentrate and handle boredom and stress. He envies those people who still wear strappies, especially when he is enjoying a few drinks. He feels left out when all his friends remove their strappies. He begins to hate the stigma of being a non strappie wearer.

One day he has a massive row with his girlfriend. Forgetting he is no longer a strappie wearer, she storms out the house into the garden intending to remove his strap and enjoy halving his stress. Once there, he remembers that there is no strappie to remove. This means there is no escape from his stress. He feels deprived and frustrated.

The next day he is back wearing his strappie. He is reluctant to discuss his failure to remain a non - strappie wearer. He tells you that life is just too stressful for him to manage without it. He promises that one day he will give it up for good.

You know stappie wearing is pointless but you do not judge him. You are not anti - strappie wearer. You respect his choice. You simply feel sorry for him.

It goes without saying that smoking or taking nicotine in any shape or form has no more benefit than being a strappie wearer! Once you have quit you will inevitably still see people holding cigarettes and vapes aloft in between puffs, just like the people in the strappie story hold their straps aloft whilst they are recovering from wearing them. So when you see a smoker posing with a cigarette or vape in this fashion, why not amuse yourself by changing that cigarette or vape into a tight strap using your imagination? You will no longer envy that smoker. You will not judge them. Most likely, you will simply feel sorry for them.

19 - Return to the Stadium

Does this mean you could go back to the stadium, stand on a stage in front of all 95,000 people and tell them all they died for nothing?

Absolutely.

So you go back there and stand on a stage in the middle of the crowd. You look around at all the sympathetic faces. As soon as it all goes quiet you tell them they all died for nothing. They took a risk for nothing. Their response is stunned silence.

You explain to them why nicotine is useless. It doesn't relax you, it does absolutely nothing for you. All it does is put you into withdrawal for more nicotine which non smokers never go into. 100% of the pleasure of smoking is the pleasure of coming out of that withdrawal each time you light up a new cigarette. The new cigarette re-addicts you, and so the cycle goes on.

Dead silence.

Nobody replies but deep down most of them always knew that something didn't add up. Putting a stick of leaves surrounded by white paper into your mouth, lighting it up and making in into a bonfire was never a very good idea.

One man shouts out, objecting that you are telling him he died for nothing. He admits it was risky to smoke but claims cigarettes helped him to relax. You explain to him that if cigarettes really relaxed you then people who smoked 40 cigarettes a would be twice as relaxed as those who smoked 20.

The Native American gets on the stage next to you and tells them that it's true, they all died for nothing. Nature would never be so cruel as to kill 95,000 people a year if it were natural to smoke. He reveals that the Native Americans did not inhale tobacco or become hooked. He tells the crowd that they used to smoke natural varieties of tobacco, and smoked many other drugs in preference. The way the white man adopted smoking was all a dreadful mistake.

20 - A more scientific look at why nicotine is useless

If you are not scientifically minded you might want to skip the next couple of chapters, but for those who don't object to a bit of scientific jargon there is hopefully enough evidence to convince anyone that nicotine is a pointless drug. At this stage you may be hoping there is for more scientific evidence that nicotine is useless. That's understandable because the message of this book goes against the grain of conventional wisdom. It goes against our lifelong assumptions and beliefs about smoking. This is the very reason the message cannot be compressed into a tiny pamphlet. Hopefully, by the time you have read right through the entire book you will look upon the message not as theory, but as a fact.

Graphic way of explaining why taking nicotine is pointless

I'm not a huge fan of graphs, but they happen to be a very useful way of illustrating how coming out of withdrawal is an integral component of taking many drugs. Three drugs are compared - alcohol, heroin and nicotine - in terms of the amount of pleasure or relief experienced when coming out of withdrawal.

Fig 1 (next page) shows the effect of alcohol on a typical, social drinker who drinks the same amount on four consecutive occasions.

As you can see, during each drinking bout intoxication levels steadily increase, then as the effect wears off they return back down to zero level - the level of a non drinker - until the next drinking session. In other words, the drinker gets a temporary lift over and above how non drinkers feel, then gradually falls back down to the zero level as the effect of the alcohol wears off, until the next time he or she drinks when the pleasure spike occurs again.

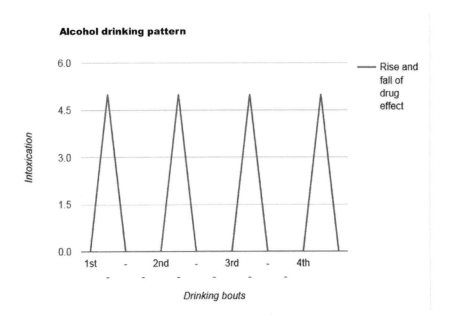

Scale on left is arbitrary representation of intoxicaton levels. The zero level (base level) represents how we normally feel when not drinking.

Please note - *scales and measurements used in these graphs are given as a rough guide and do not claim to represent any kind of experimental data.*

Fig 2 (next page) Stereotypic illustration of heroin use, assuming the user becomes quickly addicted.

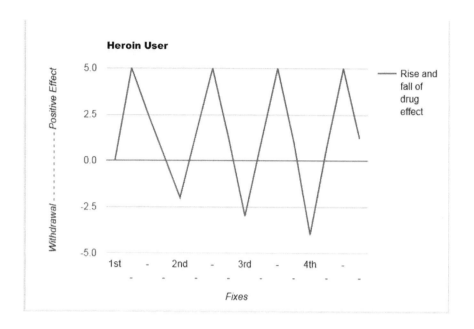

The zero level which represents how a non heroin user feels all the time - i.e. no drug effects or pleasure from heroin, but neither in withdrawal. Notice how the positive effects of each fix quickly peak then steadily fall away until the user goes into withdrawal afterwards. The next dose brings the user out of withdrawal and then takes him/her temporarily back above the zero level which represents how a non heroin user feels all the time, only to crash even further into withdrawal following each fix.

Each time the user takes heroin they plunge a little deeper into withdrawal once the effect of the drug wears off. The point being made here is that much of the "pleasure" or relief when taking drugs like heroin is actually the recovery from withdrawal. By the time of the 4th fix almost *half* the pleasure is simply due to coming out of withdrawal.

Fig 3 (below) Illustration of the drug effect of nicotine on a typical, regular smoker.

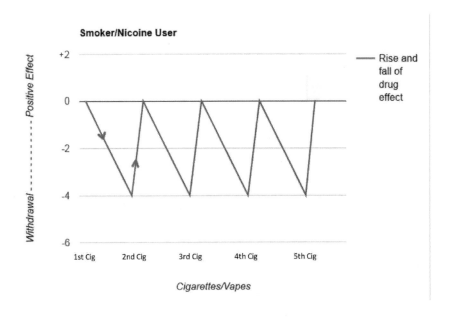

What strikes you straight away about this graph is how the zero level is at the top. The zero level represents how a non smoker (someone who never experiences nicotine withdrawal) feels all day long. You can clearly see that the smoker never goes above the level of a non smoker. Nicotine is the only one out of the three drugs compared where the effect of the drug starts in a *downward* direction.

This graph illustrates how, in contrast to heroin, the pleasure from nicotine comes purely from the experience of resurfacing from withdrawal back up to the level non smoker - in other words, up to the level that non smokers are experiencing all the time.

The downward arrow show the fall into withdrawal, after stubbing out, as nicotine is excreted from the body. The upward arrow shows the subsequent rise, or positive effect of nicotine, on smoking the next cigarette, during which period the smoker can feel a massive wave of relief and pleasure. However, it can be clearly seen that the smoker simply rises to the level of the non smoker for brief spikes. After each new cigarette or vape, the smoker/nicotine user slides steadily back into withdrawal as the fresh dose is excreted from the body.

This final graph tells you everything you need to know about why smoking is useless. It does not appear in the early stages of this book because if you show it to people too early on in the process some of them simply wince with disbelief!

21 - Doesn't the brain release pleasure hormones when we smoke?

In the age of the internet anyone can go online and quickly discover that conventional scientific wisdom assumes (as most people do) that nicotine provides pleasure. Hardly surprising then, that when people learn that the brain produces pleasure neurotransmitters such as dopamine during smoking, they challenge the notion that nicotine is a useless drug.

Nicotine, like many addictive drugs, attaches to the core neurons of the brain's reward system in **the ventral tegmental area,** where essential behaviors such as drinking water are rewarded. These neurons trigger the release of the neurotransmitter dopamine in a nearby area called the **nucleus accumbens**. When nicotine enters the body these neurons increase their activity, flooding the nucleus accumbens with dopamine, which produces pleasure and a disposition to repeat the behaviors that led to the dopamine release.

The crucial thing to understand is that these neurotransmitters are only released to reward the user for *replenishing* nicotine! Bear in mind that the brain also releases reward neurotransmitters when we replenish non drug substances such as FOOD and WATER.

Reward circuits in the brain make us enjoy eating. If we didn't eat, we wouldn't survive, so all kinds of neurotransmitters are released, such as Dopamine, once food has been swallowed. The same goes for water, and the longer we go without food or water the greater the neurochemical reward once food and water are ingested. Food and water are not necessarily absorbed into the blood stream, nor do they need to be in order for the reward circuits to be triggered - they simply need to be consumed.

The same thing appears to happens with nicotine. Unlike food and water, nicotine is not essential for our survival but for whatever reason, once we smoke regularly, the brain treats it as if it is essential, or at least beneficial to the body. *As soon as droplets of nicotine arrive in the lungs,* the reward circuits are triggered. It does not even seem to be necessary for nicotine to arrive in the brain in order for this to happen. It takes a minimum of 7 seconds for nicotine to reach the brain after inhalation, often considerably longer, and yet as any smoker will testify, the feelings of relief peak and are felt simultaneously with each drag. There is no need to wait.

During smoking nicotine levels in the brain steadily rise (Rose et al 2010). Levels do not rise and fall in correspondence to inhalation and pauses between puffs as was previously believed. In other words, there is no spike in brain levels of nicotine during inhalation. Despite this, pleasure during smoking most definitely peaks during inhalation and falls away during pauses - despite the fact that nicotine levels are continuing to rise in the brain during pauses - strongly suggesting that the brain's reward mechanism is activated by ingestion of the drug into the body rather than through delivery to the brain.

Amazingly, nicotine levels in the brain can continue to rise briefly *after* a smoker has stubbed out. In contrast to this, pleasure levels drop rapidly once the smoker stops inhaling and finishes the cigarette. This is the greatest evidence of all that it is not the presence of nicotine in the brain that is causing the reward circuits to release pleasure hormones, but rather the quantity of nicotine ingested by the body, just as is the case with food and water.

Remember, nicotine is a purely stimulant drug

Therefore there is no neurochemical rational that nicotine should have sedating effect or alleviate stress. This is demonstrated by the complete absence of any such effect on smoking the first cigarette or taking the first nicotine dose. However, once the smoker is addicted and is experiencing experience withdrawal symptoms between doses of nicotine, the brain releases dopamine and other natural neurotransmitters as a reward simply for replenishing the drug.

It doesn't help when psychologists make statements such as: "Nicotine activates the brain circuitry that regulates feelings of pleasure" or "Nicotine creates an immediate sense of relaxation." Those kind of statements are very misleading because, as mentioned, food and water, which are not drugs, do the same thing. Like nicotine, they activate brain circuitry that regulates feelings of pleasure.

If the chemical action of nicotine brought about "feelings of pleasure", why is it that smoking 40 cigarettes a day rather than 20 doesn't double those feelings?" Why is it that heavy smokers are not constantly on a high from enjoying "feelings of pleasure?" Why is it that the more people smoke the more anxious they become? Why is it that almost universally, the first ever cigarette provides no "feelings of pleasure" whatsoever? And how do they account for the fact that pleasure is experienced even before nicotine even reaches the brain?

Nesbitts paradox

Most scientists, doctors and psychologists are hopelessly confused by nicotine. They simply can't understand why chemically nicotine is 100% a stimulant drug and yet appears to also act as a sedative - a drug that relaxes you. This apparent dual action is sometimes referred to as "Nesbitt's Paradox." Named after Paul Nesbitt (1969) who attempted to fathom out how smoking appears to simultaneously soothe stress but enhances alertness.

Professor Andy Parrott of Swansea University (1998) argued there was no paradox at all, stating that nicotine *is* simply a stimulant drug. In Parrott's words, the relaxant properties of nicotine is purely the relief of irritability which develops between cigarettes.

He claimed that Nesbitt's Paradox is therefore not actually a paradox, and was never was a paradox. According to Parrott, smoking isn't about seeking pleasure but about satisfying a brain "wanting" disorder.

22 - Proving that nicotine is a useless from different angles

As mentioned earlier, all good theories should be provable from not just one angle, but several...so here they are:

1. **Doubling up the dose**. If nicotine genuinely relaxed you then doubling up the amount you smoke or vape in a day should make you twice as relaxed.

It doesn't.

Smoking 20 cigarettes a day doesn't make you twice as relaxed as when you smoke 10 a day. People who smoke 40 cigarettes a day are not twice as relaxed as people who smoke 20 a day. People who smoke 80 a day are not twice as relaxed as those who smoke 40. Think about it - the 80 a day man or woman is probably the most unsettled, edgy, nervous dude you ever met in your life! The people who smoke most heavily are the most nervy people on the planet because they are full of a useless stimulant - nicotine. Not only that, there is so much stimulant in their bodies their blood pressure is usually off the scale!

2. **The first cigarette.** If the pleasure from smoking or vaping arises solely from the elimination of withdrawal for nicotine then the first ever cigarette should provide no pleasure from a drug point of view.

It doesn't.

The only exception being the rare circumstance when someone is already addicted to nicotine because of passive smoking, or smoking spliffs.

3. **Non Smokers**. If nicotine really provided pleasure and relaxation smokers should be more relaxed, less anxious and better able to cope with life than non smokers.

They aren't.

A massive survey of around 6,500 people showed that smokers are *twice* as anxious and depressed as non smokers. Not only that, but once they have managed to quit for a year levels fall to about the same as non smokers (West 2015). That is pretty powerful evidence that Smoking is bad for the mind as well as the body!

4. **Binge Smoking.** If cigarettes relaxed you or lifted you, then smoking several in a row should produce a steady increase in pleasure, give a greater buzz or a higher lift.

This does not happen.

Unlike other drugs such as alcohol, cocaine, crystal meth, cannabis, LSD or heroin where a

greater dose gives you a greater effect, increasing nicotine dose does not increase the effect at all, in fact the opposite happens. This is because the effect isn't coming from the drug itself, it is coming solely from the relief of withdrawal symptoms that build up between doses. If insufficient time is given for withdrawal to accrue, there is little or no withdrawal to eliminate and therefore the pleasure *decreases* rather than increases. The more cigarettes that are smoked in a row, the less pleasure is experienced with each cigarette. In fact, the shorter the interval between any two cigarettes, the less pleasure will be noticed - which is why heavy smokers get progressively less pleasure the more they smoke.

5. **Double length cigarettes**. If cigarettes really relaxed you then double length ones would be available to provide double the relaxation.

They don't even exist.

They do not exist for the same reason, as given above, that binge smoking leads to a steady *decrease* in pleasure rather than an increase. Otherwise there would surely have been a market at some time historically, somewhere in the world for longer, bigger cigarettes, just as there is a market for double sized drinks - but they have never existed.

6. **The returning cigarette.** Many smokers manage to quit successfully for a considerable time, avoiding nicotine in any shape or form, only to succumb and return to smoking months or years later. When they finally light up again they are anticipating a huge pleasure, but...

It's a disappointment.

Anyone who has ever returned to smoking (if they are honest) will tell you that the first cigarette is a huge disappointment. Often the lead up to this coveted, returning cigarette will be months or years of envying those who still smoke, fantasising about the pleasure of cigarettes, recalling the enjoyment they used to experience. Eventually when they finally give in and have one, it does nothing for them - at least not from a drug point of view.

Why?

This is because the returning cigarette is in many ways identical to the first ever cigarette in that there are no withdrawal symptoms from nicotine to be eradicated. Therefore the brain gives no reward for replenishing nicotine. Remember, the whole pleasure of smoking comes from relieving the withdrawal symptoms for nicotine, therefore there is no pleasure from the returning cigarette.

Returning smokers are often surprised, confused, or disappointed that they obtain no pleasure from that cigarette, especially as they likely to be only too aware that by smoking again they will have re-addicted themselves. Sometimes they follow it up by smoking several others in quick succession, desperate to rediscover the old pleasure or drown their sorrows for having made such a rash move. The old pleasure does not take long to return however, this is of course because nicotine is a very quickly addictive drug and the returning cigarette will have re-addicted them, which means that shortly afterwards they will go back into withdrawal. Subsequent cigarettes thereafter remove the fresh withdrawal symptoms and the familiar relief followed by sinking back into withdrawal between each cigarette, or vape, returns with a vengeance.

7. **Champix** (Chantix/Varenicline Tartrate).

The goal of the anti-smoking drug Champix is to help the smoker quit by blocking nicotine receptors in the brain and therefore, theoretically, making smoking pleasure impossible. The drug was launched amid lots of excitement. It certainly succeeded in blocking the nicotine receptors, but...

People carried on smoking anyway!

The whole rationale behind drugs like Champix is flawed because it is based on the common assumption that nicotine, as a drug, provides pleasure. If the pharmacological effect of nicotine was to cause a feeling of pleasure you'd expect higher levels of nicotine in the brain to produce increased levels of pleasure....but they don't! Nicotine levels reach a maximum about 5 minutes after lighting up (Rose et al 2010) and yet a smoker gets the greatest sense of relief and pleasure at the start of a cigarette when brain levels are very low. The pleasure diminishes towards the end of the cigarette, just as, ironically, nicotine levels in the brain are peaking! PET scans have shown that drawing in smoke does NOT produce spikes of nicotine levels in the brain, and yet it is when drawing smoke in, and holding it in the lungs, that the smoker typically report the greatest pleasure.

This suggests that the pleasure from smoking does not corresponds to nicotine delivery to the brain. Instead, reward neurotransmitters are released (and pleasure felt) as nicotine *is ingested into the body*, usually by the lungs, in the same way they are released as a reward for ingesting food and water. In fact the very same centre in the brain releases reward hormones for nicotine, food and water alike. Water is not a drug, yet the brain releases neurotransmitters as a reward when water supplies are replenished, even as the liquid is being swallowed. In other words, the brain rewards us simply for topping up nicotine within the body, just as it does when we top up food and water.

This is why Champix failed to cure the world of smoking. The purpose of Champix is to block nicotine receptors in the brain. Regardless of the degree to which this is achieved, smokers continue to get pleasure because the drug does not prevent nicotine from being ingested by the body. Champix was first launched under much clamour and excitement because it was believed by many that the drug might end smoking addiction completely because it prevented the brain's pleasure centres from receiving nicotine. As I have suggested, the whole rationale behind drugs like Champix is flawed because it is based on the assumption that nicotine, as a drug, provides pleasure.

The most likely reason Champix ever works at all is the placebo effect (belief that the drug will work rather than because of any pharmaceutical action). It is also one of the world's most deadly medicines - killing more people who take it each year than any other prescription drug.

8. NicVax.

In 2005 a vaccine was developed that could stop nicotine uptake in the brain. As with Champix, the expectation was that if the brain could no longer receive nicotine the smoker would no longer get any pleasure and would no longer wish to smoke. The hope was it would cure the world of smoking!

It failed completely.

Results from clinical studies showed that smokers injected with the vaccine were no more likely to stop than those given a placebo! Not surprisingly, the company making the vaccine went bust.

This really had scientists scratching their brains. They had managed to find a substance which stopped nicotine reaching the brain and yet still smokers weren't quitting!

Like the Champix failure, it provides further evidence that the brain releases neurotransmitters when nicotine is ingested by the body, *as a reward for replenishing the drug*, not when it reaches the brain. In much the same way, for example, as it releases pleasure when quenching thirst for example. Water is not a drug, yet the brain releases neurotransmitters as water supplies are replenished, in fact, even as the liquid is being swallowed.

It seems therefore that the very presence of nicotine as a substance within the body is *indirectly* bringing about the release of pleasure hormones, not because of the pharmacological effect nicotine has as a drug.

There are new nicotine vaccines being developed but they will all fail for the same reason. Even of nicotine molecules are destroyed before they reach the brain the pleasure of smoking will still occur.

23 - Food, water, air, nicotine

If nicotine provides no benefit as a drug - why does the brain (or body) produce nicotine withdrawal?

Once you understand that nicotine is a completely useless drug and that by becoming a non smoker you are making no sacrifice whatsoever, do withdrawal symptoms simply disappear? Unfortunately it's not that simple. That's because it isn't *you* who is in charge of the craving. That craving or desire to smoke is coming from a much deeper, unconscious process within the mind or body. Whether you believe smoking to be an addiction or just a habit, once you become a regular smoker, the desire to smoke is out of your hands, it is controlled by a deeper, automatic process and you become "programmed to smoke". The overwhelming desire or craving to smoke does not occur in non smokers because they are not programmed to smoke. Some people ask an obvious question. If nicotine does nothing for the mind or body why is it an addictive drug? Why do we experience withdrawal pangs and symptoms once nicotine has been excreted from the body?

To understand this you have to understand the very source of the cravings. No one knows for sure why any addiction is produced by the mind or body. Obviously, we know that few people can deliberately or consciously switch off the desire to smoke (the craving for nicotine), it occurs automatically as nicotine levels in the body diminish, so it's out of our conscious control.

One process we cannot override is the survival mechanism within the mind and body. It is constantly monitoring levels of essential ingredients for your body. It knows that the primary things you need on a constant basis are:

FOOD, WATER AND AIR

It monitors the amount of food coming in and if levels of food run low it will make you hungry, if your body is low on liquid it will make you thirsty, if you do not breathe it will eventually force you to breathe. Food, water and air, that's basically what it thinks you need everyday - and its right, without these things you will die. You cannot switch off this powerful programming, you are born with it, and it is far too important for you to be allowed a conscious override. It is unbelievably powerful.

If you like, hunger is a withdrawal symptom of not having sufficient food, thirst is a withdrawal symptom of insufficient water and the sensation of suffocation is a withdrawal symptom of insufficient air.

Food water and air, that's all you basically need. But what if the brain were to add a completely useless forth item to that list, something totally useless to the mind or body? Then where would you be? What would happen if it added *nicotine* to that essential list?

FOOD, WATER , AIR *and* NICOTINE

Well then it would produce a craving for nicotine just as soon as nicotine levels went down beyond a certain point. You would be programmed to smoke. And that seems to be more or less exactly what happens. In other words, the brain doesn't think it would be *nice* for you to smoke, it's as if it believes that nicotine is essential for your survival.

Once the brain is programmed to regard nicotine as an essential ingredient for the human body it calls for nicotine regularly regardless of your mood or state of mind. It makes us feel uneasy as levels get lower, as if nicotine was like a vital fatty acid, or a vitamin or something else essential for our continued survival. It does not even care what the drug does to you, whether it relaxes you, stimulates you or anything else for that matter. It just believes that the substance must be kept topped up within the body to a given level. This explains why it is so hard to give up smoking.

Ironically, it is only trying to *help* you. It is not a "Monster" within you. It seems more likely to me that your brain is actually trying to *help* you by producing the craving.

Remember nicotine is a totally useless substance, it is a deadly poison that has absolutely no use or function whatsoever. As a drug, when administered for the first time it produces no feeling of elation, euphoria, satisfaction, relaxation or any other mental or physical benefit...these sensations are only produced in response to recovery from withdrawal from the drug.

Once your brain notices that you have not smoked for some time, say overnight, it produces a much greater desire for you to smoke, or an increased level of withdrawal symptoms such as the inability to concentrate or relax. The part of the brain monitoring nicotine levels becomes concerned that levels of the drug have fallen and remained low for some time, just as it becomes concerned if water or nutrients levels in the body remain low. Of course you can continue through the day and ignore these symptoms, but eventually you are bound to give in and light up a cigarette, and once a sufficient amount of nicotine is being replenished the brain removes all the withdrawal symptoms. Nearly all smokers assume that the pleasant feeling that ensues is a boost due to the action of nicotine, but we know that cannot be so because no such boost pleasant feeling is experienced the first time the drug is taken.

If nicotine delivery fails for 2 or 3 days the brain battles hard to get you to smoke. Remember it is the survival function that is monitoring nicotine levels. It doesn't care whether the drug relaxes you, stimulates you or does anything else - it just wants nicotine replenished because it is convinced it is an essential for he body, almost as if it thinks you will die without nicotine.... no wonder so many languages share the phrase:

"I'm dying for a cigarette"

The brain and body know that nicotine has been coming in sometimes for years, that it gets distributed all over the body, and is used to that balance. It seems as if the brain regards the presence of nicotine as the "correct" balance, the normal homeostasis. It could be that the brain is trying to get nicotine topped out to redress a homeostatic imbalance that occurs as soon as it is excreted from the body - after all we know that regulation of food intake relies on communication between reward and homeostatic neurocircuits. Once nicotine is excreted, that balance changes and the brain and body call for its replenishment by producing a niggle to smoke, then a need, then a craving.

In other words you are up against your body's own survival mechanism – no wonder it can be so hard to quit. The longer you "deprive" your body of nicotine the worse you feel. If you are a strong willed person who prides themselves on your determination and will power you may wonder why you find it so hard to stay quit.

In fact, the brain may be confusing nicotine with a substance known as acetylcholine that *is* essential to the body. It's a neurotransmitter that has a very similar molecular similarity to nicotine. Nicotine locks to the same sensors in the brain as acetylcholine. When this happens, the whole system then gets confused, and as if it now has a corrupted computer disc the brain steadily calls for more and more nicotine to be present.

In a way you are up against yourself. The mind has often been compared to an iceberg, the conscious mind, the bit we think with and have control over, is only the tip of the iceberg. Beneath the surface is the subconscious mind, much larger, more powerful and hidden. It can do a lot of good, but if wrongly programmed can unwittingly do us a lot of harm. The more powerful your conscious mind (i.e. your will power to stop the intake of nicotine), the more powerful your subconscious mind (i.e. the automatic process that regards nicotine as essential for survival). Rather than doing battle with a monster within you, by stopping smoking you are ignoring and overriding a process that is actually trying to do the very best it can for you. It is producing the cravings with the very best intentions.

I believe it only leaves you alone when it is quite sure of two things:

1. That the drug nicotine is, in fact, completely useless and unnecessary for both the mind and body.

2. That you will never ever smoke or take nicotine in any shape or form ever again.

Once this mechanism goes without nicotine for a week or two physical withdrawal symptoms usually disappear. This is because this mechanism then realises or learns that nicotine, far from being essential to you, is quite unnecessary. It is quite capable of then switching off all desire and craving and leaving you alone.

Car headrest analogy

These days car computers are very sophisticated. You will see a warning light, not just when fuel is running low but also if there is insufficient oil, and even when there is not enough air in the tyres. Just suppose they invent a special kind of car headrest, fitted with a device that actually starts prodding you when you start running low on fuel. The lower the fuel gets the more frequent and intense the prodding becomes - prompting you to visit a garage and fill up. Not only that but it taps your left shoulder if you are low on oil, scratches your back if you are low on water, and flicks your ear if tyre pressure is low. It really is a very clever device.

But something goes wrong. You're driving along and it starts to prod your neck, even though you have just filled up with petrol. You soon begin to feel very uncomfortable and irritated. It prods you all day long and in the end you visit your garage and ask them to fix it, but the mechanic sees a purple light flashing on the dashboard and tells you the prodding is because the car computer is telling you that you are low on diesel. You explain that it is a petrol car and doesn't need diesel, but the mechanic keeps telling you you need diesel.

You ask to speak to the manager, who apologises and explains that the car's computer is only trying to help you by prodding you to fill up with diesel. There is a mistake in the programming and it doesn't realise the car does not need diesel. They try to reprogramme the computer but he disc is write protected.

However the manager informs you it won't matter because it is an ingenious, self learning computer. Over the next few days it will gradually stop prodding your neck as it works out that the car does not come to a halt without diesel. Sure enough after about 4 days the computer notices that the car functions perfectly without diesel and the prodding steadily fades and then stops completely.

The human brain can behave in a similar way when you quit smoking. It's as if there is a computer in there that is monitoring the amount of nicotine that comes into your body. Nicotine is non essential to the human body and as a drug it is completely useless, but the brain doesn't seem to be aware of this. When levels become low or "nicotine tanks" are empty it keeps producing a desire, or craving to smoke or vape. If you ignore it long enough, the brain re-programs and it leaves you alone. It steadily learns that nicotine is not essential to you at all.

This is why it's important to let the message that nicotine is useless to go as deep as possible. The more your brain understands the message the easier it will be when you quit.

24 - Ironically, Smoking Causes Stress

Smokers typically claim that cigarettes help relieve feelings of stress and that mood control was an important reason for smoking. However, surveys show that the stress level of adult smokers is much higher than those of non smokers. A study that looked at stress and smoking in hospital nurses (Tagliacozzo 1982) found significantly higher scores for smokers than for non-smokers on scales concerning the physical and emotional stress of the job and the dissatisfaction with its rewards.

A study of nearly 6,500 people over the age of 40 found that smokers are almost *twice* as likely to suffer from anxiety and depression. Not only that but quitting was shown to reverse the situation - just a year after they quit, smokers anxiety levels were virtually the same as non-smokers (West 2015).

Dr Andy Parrott, an authority on human psychobiology, looked at more than 30 international studies examining the relationship between smoking and stress (1999). He found that the stress levels of adult smokers was slightly higher than those of non smokers. The studies also showed that adolescent smokers experience increasing levels of stress as they develop regular patterns of smoking. Surveys also found that when smokers mange to quit smoking they gradually become less stressed over time.

To quote Parrott:

"Far from acting as an aid for mood control, nicotine dependency seems to exacerbate stress. This is confirmed in the daily mood patterns described by smokers, with normal moods during smoking and worsening moods between cigarettes. Thus, the apparent relaxant effect of smoking only reflects the reversal of the tension and irritability that develop during nicotine depletion. Dependent smokers need nicotine to remain feeling normal. The message that tobacco use does not alleviate stress but actually increases it needs to be far more widely known. It could help those adult smokers who wish to quit and might prevent some school children from starting."

Smoking makes you moody.

Many smokers find their mood fluctuate depending upon the length of time since their last cigarette. In between cigarettes the withdrawal symptoms for nicotine increase and even light smokers can become nervous, snappy or irritable when nicotine levels are low. A smoker will typically become noticeably more cheerful in anticipation of the next cigarette, which temporarily relieves the withdrawal symptoms. In contrast to this, once the cigarette is being stubbed out the smoker is left feeling slightly lethargic, jaded and subdued due to the combined effect of reduced oxygen, plus the poisoning effect of nicotine and other ingredients.

25 - Occasional or light smokers

O
ccasional or light smokers are either immune to the addictive nature of nicotine, or are far less addicted. However, without becoming properly addicted they cannot obtain the huge feeling of relief that occurs when coming out of nicotine withdrawal. Unlike regular smokers they are much more prone to noticing the light headed feelings and sensations of increased body heaviness that sometime go with smoking. As soon as nicotine reaches the bloodstream it reduces the ability of haemoglobin to transport oxygen to the brain which causes these feeling of light headedness to occur in first time and occasional smokers. The effect is far less easily noticed, if at all, by regular and heavy smokers.

Some occasional smokers, however, *are* mildly addicted to nicotine. They are usually unaware that the occasional, overwhelming desire to smoke is due to the need to eliminate nicotine withdrawal, which has been slowly increasing in the background since their last cigarette, rather than their choice to indulge occasionally in what appears to be a relaxing or uplifting experience. They are unaware that after stubbing out the cigarette or cigarettes smoked on a single occasion, they will begin to steadily go into withdrawal for nicotine over the days following the cigarette.

Let's say, for example, a woman tries her first ever cigarette. Like most people, she is not much impressed from a drug point of view. She may find the smoke a little unpleasant but is aware that this aversion to the poison of tobacco can be overcome by persistence and experience. She soon notices a feeling of being light headed and may even assume, incorrectly, that this is the pleasure of smoking that she has witnessed so many smokers enjoying in the past - but she is unimpressed by it.

Like virtually all first time smokers she is underwhelmed and not impressed. She assumes that she will never become hooked. Her dislike of cigarettes encourages her to feel she may allow herself to smoke occasionally as a social prop, after all smoking is a symbol of maturity, independence and toughness.

She becomes an occasional smoker, and smokes a cigarette or two with a smoker friend on Friday night, and then does not have another one till the following Friday. On Saturday morning she awakens feeling a little dejected, irritable, below par, or simply feels slightly less happy than usual. She puts it down to the stresses of life, to fluctuations in her mood, health, tiredness or even to pure chance, not realising she is increasingly experiencing the subtle withdrawal symptoms for nicotine, which will increase a little more each day. By Monday she is feeling increasingly stressed but does her best to put the feelings into the background.

The following Friday she is still experiencing the slight nicotine withdrawal in the background, but is unaware of what it is. She meets the same smoker friend and has her first cigarette in an entire week. As soon as she begins inhaling the smoke she begins to come out of nicotine withdrawal and in a matter of seconds. All the withdrawal symptoms accumulated over the last

week evaporate - giving her a feeling of elation and pleasure. She assumes the pleasant feeling is down to the properties within the drug nicotine, not realising the drug is incapable of causing any positive feelings, the pleasure is caused simply by the elimination of the withdrawal symptoms. The next time she meets the same smoker friend she is even more addicted and is therefore very much hoping she will again be offered a cigarette again - and so the addictive cycle continues. At this point some occasional smokers refrain from buying their own cigarettes but most go on to become fully fledged smokers.

Many occasional smokers are basically serial quitters without realising it. Instead of having another cigarette, say the day after, to bring them out of the mild withdrawal that follows each occasional cigarette, they simply endure it for several days either until it eventually fades away, in much the same way as it does after someone quits, or more likely, until they meet up with friends who smoke and have another cigarette. As I have said, they have no idea are experiencing very mild nicotine withdrawal after each smoking session, and put the feelings down to just going through a difficult patch in the day, a natural downturn, tiredness, a period of nervousness or mood fluctuations.

If they go long enough between cigarettes the withdrawal will have faded away by time they light it up again, therefore they won't get the kick that regular smokers get from coming out of withdrawal. If, as is more likely, some of the withdrawal remains, they will get the very pleasant relief of eliminating the remaining withdrawal - they will feel as if they are emerging from the downturn, from the difficult patch!

The slippery slope

In the initial stages the occasional smoker can carry on having one cigarette a week, say on a social occasion. In the days between each cigarette they continue to experience mild nicotine withdrawal each time but barely notice it. Like all smokers they are not as calm and as relaxed as they were before they smoked but they put this down to maybe just going through difficult time in life.

They can carry on smoking in this manner for some time, but then, let's say for example, the occasional smoker gets into an argument with someone and has not had a cigarette for a few days. Once again, a substantial amount of the unpleasant stressful feelings they are experiencing and their inability to cope is actually due to nicotine withdrawal, which has been silently accumulating since the last cigarette a few days ago. As always, they have no idea of this and have barely noticed the increase in stress caused by drug withdrawal. The other half of the half of the stress is due to the actual argument itself. The light smoker decides to have a cigarette and by doing so quickly removes the 50% of unpleasant feeling that is purely nicotine withdrawal and therefore halve their stress! They then feel better able to handle the real life stress.

In this way light smokers conclude that smoking helps with stress. Subsequently when, inevitably, they have another bad day or difficult period in their life in the future they are likely to turn to cigarettes. Withdrawal means they will be feeling down more frequently anyway, which adds to the increased likelihood they will begin to smoke more often.

Of course if they smoke too frequently, they are not going enough time between cigarettes for much withdrawal to accumulate. When any smokers decides to smoke much more than usual or binge smoke, it therefore does not continue to provide pleasure or relieve stress because insufficient withdrawal has accumulated. Chasing pleasure in this way always fails. This puzzles the binge smoker because if they increase the amount of just about any other recreational drug, say alcohol or cocaine, the pleasure increases proportionately. All that is achieved by taking in more nicotine than normal is that they become much more addicted and the brain then subsequently calls for nicotine more frequently. This means the desire to smoke begins to occur at much more frequent intervals and the occasional smoker is now on the slippery slope to becoming a heavier smoker. This does not happen through choice but rather through addiction. The reality is they now are compelled to smoke more frequently because withdrawal is accumulating more quickly and more deeply.

You could not invent a more devious trap.

All smokers start off as occasional smokers but it is a usually a slippery slope towards becoming an every day smoker. Only a small percentage of people who start smoking as teenagers remain being occasional smokers and never go on to become heavier smokers. These are probably the ones who are not hooked on nicotine because of their physiological makeup.

Incidentally it is impossible for anyone who has gone on to become an every day smoker (in other words a full blown smoking addict) to cut down and return to being an occasional, or even a light smoker. This is because smoking addiction is very like alcohol addiction and heroin addiction - rather like a ratchet or cog in a machine that can only go in one direction. In over twenty years of helping people quit smoking I have never met a regular smoker who went back to being an occasional smoker.

How to quit if you are an occasional smoker

As mentioned earlier, some occasional smokers appear to be physiologically immune to the addictiveness of nicotine. The only effects they will likely ever experience when smoking are light headedness, coupled sometimes with a feeling of bodily heaviness, and the mild stimulant affect of nicotine such as an increase in blood pressure.

If you fit into this category and enjoy those feelings there is a way you can obtain them, or at least something similar, without smoking. All you need do is hold your breath for a minute or so and you will begin to feel light headed without smoking at all! If you were to couple this with a dose of caffeine, from say tea or coffee, then you can simultaneously mimic the mild stimulant effect of nicotine.

So next time you are out drinking with friends and fancy one of your rare cigarettes, simply retreat from the company you are in. Hold your breath for a minute or so then rejoin your friends. Your body will likely feel different, slightly heavier than usual and you will experience that familiar light headedness. Sip on a tea or coffee and there you are...as a good as a cigarette!

Please note, holding breath can be hazardous for some people, so you do this at your own risk! Also, this will only work for occasional or light smokers. It won't work so well for regular or heavy smokers however, because they get an entirely different pleasure from smoking. They rarely notice the light headed feeling at all and as described many times already in this book, they obtain their pleasure from relieving the withdrawal symptoms that crop up gradually between each cigarette.

26 - The Hardened Smoker

Deep down, virtually all smokers know that smoking is pointless, but there is always the odd exception - those smokers who still believe that smoking has a benefit, regardless of any danger. Hardened smoker often fall into this category but they are not necessarily heavy smokers - some are light or occasional smokers.

Whether you count yourself as a hardened smoker or not, it's worthwhile reading this chapter because some of the things that prevent hardened smokers from stopping may also be stopping you.

Committed smokers, especially chain smokers, get easily irritated and defensive at the slightest mention of quitting, and they are generally well practiced in the art of self defence. When a hardened smoker is resentful of those who warn them of the dangers, it is reminiscent of the king who wants to shoot the messenger. On the other hand, there is nothing more hypocritical than an ex-smoker who takes a delight in lecturing those who still smoke! Actually, I believe in respecting people's choice to smoke. I dislike the way heavy smokers are pilloried by society.

Confirmed smokers who refuse to stop (or more likely have repeatedly failed to stop) sometimes say they would rather take the risks. They will tell you things like it's "one of the little things that make life worth living." Their typical argument for smoking is "why spend your life worrying when you might be run over by a bus tomorrow?" My answer to that would be to ask them how many people run over by a bus can you fit into Wembley Stadium every year? I'd imagine that the number is probably in single figures. You would barely notice them if they walked onto the pitch, but you would certainly notice the 95,000 who died from smoking.

They counter this by saying the damage they have already done to their lungs and body is probably irreversible anyway so they might as well carry on smoking. After all, they enjoy smoking and as they say, a shorter, sweeter life well lived is better than a longer one spent feeling deprived.

They are usually surprised when I then tell them I am not remotely anti smoker. As I have repeated many times in this book, I am not anti drug taking, after all, drinking alcohol, tea, coffee or Coca Cola are all forms of drug taking. I am pro freedom and pro individual choice - it's just that smoking is pointless from a drug point of view.

When I go on to say that if I believed nicotine could provide true enjoyment, or had any benefit whatsoever *from a drug point of view* I might even smoke or vape myself - regardless of all the well known dangers - that usually gets their attention. As you will hear in the next chapter I wouldn't smoke again even if there was a safe cigarette, purely because nicotine has no benefit whatsoever as a drug.

The truth is, most hardened smokers see smoking as a pleasure or crutch they cannot live without. They believe smoking to be completely natural, a right, and feel comforted and supported by the fact that until recently most adults smoked, and that even now, they are reassuringly surrounded by the one in five adults who still smoke. Actually, almost everyone assumes that smoking is natural, not realising that inhaling tobacco smoke into the lungs was not practiced by natives who gave us tobacco in the first place. Some committed smokers will go to any extreme in order to stay in denial of the health risks, but others, though fully aware of the dangers, seem to possess a kind of courageous, wartime spirit. After all, danger never prevented people from putting on a brave face and remaining cheerful.

They assume they would never be able to enjoy life without smoking. They believe life would be second rate without it and they would never feel as confident in social occasions. They would lose a useful crutch, a friend, a means of concentrating, a way of releasing their creativity or handling stress. When they have attempted to quit before they have failed. They have likely felt bereaved, totally unable to cope. They have missed smoking badly, they have endured persistent longings and cravings, they have envied all those who still smoke, for example when drinking or having a break.

Quite often they readily admit they are addicted, but assume it is an addiction to a drug that benefits them. If they hear anything to the contrary they immediately assume it must be some kind of cranky message, or a play on words thought up by the anti-pleasure brigade, the politically correct, or the nanny state. Even if you spell it out clearly to them why nicotine use is pointless, it's as if they cannot take in what is being said. Like telling someone who has been in a cage for many years that all along the cage door has been unlocked - they can't even begin to believe you, so they simply humour you and remain in the pointless cage.

Their basic reasoning is something like this - they find an immense release of stress at times when they smoke, & believe that smoking has genuinely helped them, at certain difficult times in their lives. Although dangerous, smoking appears to provide a crutch and a boost that non smokers do not get. It appears to give you an edge.

Whatever you tell them they simply don't truly believe that there is nothing to be gained from smoking. If true, it would mean that civilised man has been making a terrible mistake for five centuries, and besides, it is not a message they will ever likely have heard from doctors or by the mainstream media. It would mean that kings, queens, presidents, Hollywood stars and rock stars alike were all conned by tobacco. It's difficult for them to believe that every human being whoever smoked in history was simply in a trap and got absolutely no benefit from smoking whatsoever. They believe that the message that smoking is pointless amounts to nothing more than some kind of brainwashing from "do-gooder" health campaigners - not realising that the real brainwashing took place long before they even started smoking. As children we are all brainwashed by watching other people apparently getting an advantage out of smoking.

Is it that hardened smokers value cigarettes so highly they see them as indispensable? Or is it because when they try to quit they cannot endure the withdrawal and are simply resigned to their fate? Successful quitters often reassure them that once you quit you get to a point where you just don't need cigarettes or nicotine anymore, but they just don't believe that they are personally capable of ever reaching that point themselves, because in the past, no matter how long they have held out for when quitting, they always missed cigarettes and have envied those who still smoke and in the end they have always gone back.

Not realising that withdrawal symptoms crop up in between each cigarette, hardened smokers typically assume that it is the drug nicotine itself which is relaxing them. They do not realise that the feelings of nervousness, lack of confidence or irritability that they experience are actually a result of withdrawal, and many believe themselves to be nervous individuals, for whom smoking, though dangerous, is indispensable because of the way it lifts their mood. They believe they are nervous types who need a crutch and justify this to themselves as a reason to continue taking the risks. They do not realise that it is the constant, everyday withdrawal symptoms of nicotine, that they are experiencing all day long in between cigarettes, coupled with the rise in blood pressure caused by the drug and poisoning effects of smoking that make them nervous. They conclude that without the presumed boost from nicotine they will now have to cope with life in what they regard as their true state - nervous, inadequate, lacking in confidence, strength, coping ability and resilience.

Some heavy smokers come to the conclusion that others can live without cigarettes because they are fortunate to possess a different mental makeup, that these people are simply lucky enough to have more ability to relax and cope with life naturally. This belief that they are not as relaxed as other people and are therefore much more in need of a crutch in order to handle and enjoy life, is reinforced when they attempt to live without smoking and feel deprived of the perceived benefits.

So regardless of the risks, horrors and dangers of smoking, they give in and return to cigarettes, feeling they cannot personally live without nicotine, which they view as their helper, their crutch, their friend. They may go a number of days without before giving in. They may feel bad about themselves on returning but experience tremendous relief as they recover from an episode of very deep withdrawal. This reinforces the idea in their head of the indispensable value of nicotine as a drug.

You could not invent a more subtle, pernicious and ingenious trap.

The crucial thing here is their failure is based very largely on the belief that when quitting they have made a sacrifice, they have given up something

120

useful. Hopefully this book will enable even the most diehard smoker to quit successfully, once they are fully aware that there is no sacrifice being made.

Hardened smokers don't have a basic flaw in their character - they simply do not truly believe that smoking is just a pointless trap - they simply don't realise that being a nicotine addict is as crazy and pointless as being hooked on Paracetamol.

How to give up of you are a hardened smoker

Imagine someone you dearly love becomes a Paracetamol addict. You want them to give up, but although they now understand that they are hooked on a useless drug, they still refuse, telling you that they enjoy them, and in any case, they may already have irreversible liver damage. They are cheerful and seem to be past caring, resigned to the further damage they are doing to their liver. What would you tell them? You'd probably be tempted to look them straight in the eye and tell them the real reason they won't stop is addiction! Worse still, they have got themselves hooked on a totally useless drug! You would tell them to simply throw the bottle of Paracetamol in the bin!

The truth is the only reason they would carry on is that they still don't truly believe Paracetamol cannot relax you. And if you are a hardened smoker who won't quit or thinks you can't quit, maybe it's because you still don't quite see how nicotine can be a useless drug.

If that's the case, do you really think that nature would be so cruel to kill so many people each year just because of an innocent pleasure? It is estimated a hundred million people died from smoking in the Twentieth Century - nearly as many as in all wars put together. Nature wasn't being cruel at all! Each death was sending the human race the message that we were never intended to inhale tobacco smoke. After all, the people who gave it to us, The Native American Indians, drew the smoke into their mouths, like cigar smokers, and blew it out!

27 - The Safe cigarette

S mokers and ex - smokers alike often wish there was a safe cigarette...a cigarette without any of the dangers so that they could continue to enjoy the perceived drug benefits of nicotine.

Regardless of what the tobacco industry says about the dangers of smoking being exaggerated, no tobacco company boss would want their grandchildren to smoke. In fact they are now spending a fortune trying to develop a safe cigarette, or at least a safer one. This follows increasing legislation against smoking which is a real threat to cigarette sales. Smoking is big business. Worldwide, about 5.5 trillion cigarettes are currently manufactured every year and tobacco revenue is about $770 billion. With all the scare about smoking removed, there would be a lot of money in a safe or at least safer cigarette.

Not surprisingly, the world biggest tobacco company Philip Morris is investing billions into the search for such a cigarette but this just shows how widespread the false notion that nicotine provides any benefit still is.

As I have stated before, I am not anti drug, I believe in individual freedom and freedom of choice. I am not saying that all recreational drugs are bad for you.

...but I wouldn't smoke again even if there was a safe cigarette.

Tight straps may be safe but who would wear them? If you still yearn for a safe cigarette you haven't quite understood the message. That's because the idea that nicotine has any benefit, that smoking is a useful crutch, a friendly helper is so deeply ingrained in our minds. This isn't to say that other drugs can't relax you or help with stress or give you a high. I am not denying that. Just about every other recreational drug in the world will give you something - whether it's caffeine, alcohol, cannabis, ecstasy, meth, cocaine, heroin, opium - the list is endless. There are pharmaceutical drugs that can be taken for recreation on that list too - Valium (Diazepam) for example. I'm not recommending you take any of them! Some can ruin lives or harm you. You will likely have to suffer some kind of downer after all of them in some way or other- but at least they give you something. At least they do what it says on the can. Nicotine is the only drug that gives you nothing whatsoever. It is the world's only completely pointless drug. It is unique in that it is the world's only completely useless recreational drug. Why else do you think that nature culls so many people who take it? Even the Indians didn't use it as a drug, all they did was use it to blow smoke signals towards the Gods.

Have you reached the point where you wouldn't smoke even if there was a safe cigarette?

Are you sure?

If you are not completely sure, the following NLP metaphor will almost certainly get you to that point - and hopefully even give you a laugh.

28 - Trap-eze

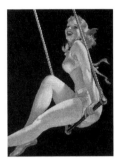

A drug doesn't have to do anything for you to get you addicted. Imagine a new drug, a recreational drug, becomes all the rage, let's call it...."Trap-eze". It's sold in capsules and looks and tastes the same as water. Trapeze works in a very unusual way. When you have the first dose it does absolutely nothing for you, nothing at all. The drug effect is completely neutral. It's pharmacological effect is just the same as water. Some people report feeling slightly light headed, the way you would if you held your breath, but that's all you notice - there is no pleasure in taking it at all.

The instructions that come with Trapeze capsules tell you that you that the drug itself will never give you a lift, but once you have taken it two or three times you will begin to go into withdrawal. Seems pointless then, but noticing how many of your friends take Trapeze on social occasions, or even thrive on them you think they must have some benefit.

A close friend tells you how she depends on Trapeze. When she feels a little stressed she has one and her stress evaporates. When she is bored she has one and all her boredom disintegrates. She has one during her morning break at work and finds that Trapeze is useful at helping her think things through, They help her to concentrate, they help her relax after food...she swears by them.

You watch your fiend taking Trapeze and from the look of relief and pleasure on her face you can see the results for yourself. You have now witnessed the drug doing all the things she claimed they could do. You decide to give them a go. You naturally want to find out what all the fuss is about.

Over the weekend you take two or three capsules from your Trapeze taking friend who knocks them back constantly. You enjoy none of them and still can't understand why they are so popular. However, on Monday morning you wake up feeling uncharacteristically low, a little below par. At first you have no idea why, then you realise are already experiencing withdrawal symptoms for the drug, just as it warned you on the packet.

Despite being able to do nothing for you Trapeze is still highly addictive. All day long at home or a work you feel slightly irritable, and can't concentrate because of the mild withdrawal

symptoms. You don't notice them so much when you are busy but when you are bored they get to you. The withdrawal seems to take a little bit of shine off everything. You don't feel as optimistic about the future, you don't wake up in the mornings feelings as fresh and as happy as you used to. You seem to have lost your old enthusiasm, your confidence, your vitality. You also notice you are feeling physically a bit below par and your skin does not look as healthy as usual.

Later in the week you meet up with the same Trapeze taking friend, but your usual sparkle seems to have disappeared and everything seems to be more of an effort than usual. The friend offers you another Trapeze, telling you it will sort you out. You hesitate, remembering how the first one did nothing for you, how it was no different to taking a capsule of water, but you go ahead and take it anyway, maybe to be sociable. Eureka! Almost straight away you notice all the withdrawal disappearing. It is a wonderful moment. All the horrible withdrawal that you have been enduring for days evaporates! As you come out of withdrawal you feel like a golden bubble. You feel lifted, your joie de vivre seems to have returned!...All thanks to Trap - eze. Of course you realise that by taking another one you have re-addicted yourself, but it was so much better than continuing to endure the withdrawal symptoms.

The drug is very quickly excreted from your body and it's only a matter of time before you begin to go back down into withdrawal. Soon you long to be free of the awful symptoms and feel normal again. You look forward to meeting your friend again in the hope that she will offer you another Trapeze. She does. You begin to hang out with that friend, and Trapeze begins to form a bond between you.

In this way you become hooked on a completely useless drug. The only pleasure it can ever give you, is the pleasure of returning to normal through removing the withdrawal symptoms. You are in a trap. That's why they call it "Trap-eze!" It only took a few doses and you were hooked. You are now a slave to a completely useless drug.

There are ads telling you that Trapeze is now available in tempting flavours like "strawberry scented", "banana split", "apple and cinnamon" just like vape juice flavours. Then to your horror, you see a TV programme that tells you Trapeze gives you cancer. Not only that it is the most carcinogenic substance in the world. It is also the biggest killer of healthy people. You learn that whether you take it once a week or all day long it makes you physically weaker, zaps your energy levels, ages your skin, gives you dark areas around your eyes, lowers your sex drive and stops you reaching your full potential as a human being. Trapeze makes you more stressed because you spend all of the time in between capsules in different states of withdrawal.

What would you do if you found yourself hooked on a completely useless drug like Trap-eze? Especially if you knew that by putting up with the mild withdrawal for a week or two would free you from the trap forever. Would you need counseling to help you? Would you chew Trapeze gum or put on a Trapeze patch? Would you start to smoke it through an electronic vapour device?..."Vap-eze?"

Of course not.

Once you are aware that a drug like Trapeze - or nicotine - is completely useless you don't need anybody to hold your hand. There are no steps to follow. Throw the drug away in the nearest bin and never touch it again!

What would be the point in a safe cigarette? If Trap-eze really existed you wouldn't take it even if it were completely safe - so what's the difference? The only way to handle the situation like being hooked on nicotine or Trap-eze is to take decisive action and quit in style.

29 - NRT and Other Drugs do Not Work

Although this book is entitled "Quit Smoking or Vaping in Style" it could just as easily have been called "Quit Nicotine in Style." This is because the basic problem we are dealing with here is not smoking or vaping, nor is it taking snuff, sucking tobacco pellets (snus) or taking nicotine in any particular form...it is *nicotine use.*

If a heroin user smokes the drug ("chasing the dragon's tail") then switches to injecting it through a needle - or some kind of transdermal heroin patch, they will have quit nothing. They will still be a heroin user - they will remain addicted to it. Likewise, for any nicotine user to claim they have quit simply because they have switched from getting the drug through a patch, gum or vapour dispenser, instead of through smoking, is complete nonsense.

As stressed in the chapter about cutting down - nicotine gum, patches and other products do not work. They do not free anyone from nicotine addiction. All they do is keep the user addicted to the drug. Every fresh dose of nicotine re-addicts the user regardless of the means by which it is delivered. Only when you stop taking nicotine can you begin to free yourself from its addiction, just like only when an alcoholic stops drinking completely can they free themselves from alcohol addiction.

Nicotine gum has now been linked with mouth and other cancer (Muy-Teck Teh et al 2009) The study cautioned the potential carcinogenic effect of nicotine in tobacco replacement therapies.

Once you have quit, it is essential that you never touch nicotine patches, gum, vapes or nicotine in any shape or form ever again. This is because they do not help anyone quit. All they do is keep you addicted to nicotine.

It's rather like offering an alcoholic an "alcohol patch" to help them give up drink! It would simply keep them addicted. Everybody knows that once you have become an alcoholic you either carry on drinking or go teetotal. If an alcoholic is giving up they can't touch even the slightest drop of alcohol ever again without going back. There is no clear definition of an alcoholic, it's simply when a drinker has gone past the stage when cutting down and reverting to lighter drinking habits has proved impossible. Once they have gone past that point they have a choice - they either continue drinking to excess every day or never touch alcohol again.

Imagine a doctor fitting an alcoholic (let's say a whiskey drinker) with a special patch or alcohol dispenser on their arm to deliver a steady drip of alcohol into the blood all day long. That would be ridiculous! Would it help? Of course not. If an alcoholic used the patch, would he or she have truly quit? No. It would produce the same results as if they sipped a few drops of whiskey from a glass all day long.

Using Nicotine Replacement Therapy (NRT) is like taking the odd puff of a cigarette or vape all day long. It simply keeps you addicted to nicotine. NRT is all complete nonsense which is why,

statistically it gives a smoker no better chance of quitting than stopping unaided. As Allen Carr once said, NRT should be called nicotine *continuation* therapy. Not surprisingly the number of people quitting successfully overall has not increased since the introduction of NRT in the early 1990s.

Research into recovery from virtually all other recreational drugs is classified according to the name of the drug concerned, e.g. abstinence from alcohol, cocaine, heroin and so on, but embarrassingly, all scientific research into NRT has historically been addressed to abstinence from "smoking" rather than nicotine - as if nicotine dependency in itself is not the problem. The addictive substance is nicotine, not smoking. The basic problem we are dealing with here isn't simply *smoking* - it is nicotine use.

NRT is now a huge industry, worth billions to drug companies worldwide. It has gained medical approval on the back of early claims that their use improves the chances of "quitting" by roughly 50%. Research statistics claim that NRT doubles your chances of quitting...but quitting what? And for how long? These statistics usually refer to quitting smoking and NOT to quitting nicotine. The nicotine user may temporarily stop getting nicotine through tobacco, i.e. smoking - but they are still getting it delivered through

NRT - so in essence they are still a nicotine user. If addicted to nicotine, they will remain so until they stop taking NRT - at which time "quit" rates become the same as those who quit unassisted.

Drug company funded trials typically only look at whether smokers have managed to avoid cigarettes for ridiculously short periods, such as six weeks, which can hardly be described as quitting! Subsequent, independent research showed that when looked at over the longer term, typically after a year, NRT results were no better than placebo or willpower:

Pierce and Gilpin (2002) analyzed data from some of the largest tobacco surveys ever conducted involving some 20,000 Californians They concluded that NRT was not effective in long term smoking cessation. Relapse rates amongst some of those on NRT was sometimes even higher than for those who quit on their own.

Then in 2010 a review of 511 studies into smoking cessation revealed that despite 20 years of NRT, the overwhelming majority of ex-smokers who successfully quit did so unaided and were twice as numerous as those who used NRT or other quit smoking drugs (Chapman and MacKenzie 2010).

A prospective study was then carried out by The Harvard School of Public Health looking at 787 smokers in Massachusetts who used different methods to quit over a 5 year period. The researchers were disappointed to find that the effectiveness of NRT was no better than using willpower - even when counseling was given to those on NRT (Hilliel Alpert et al, 2011).

The sad truth is that the initial research on NRT effectiveness was carried out by the same big pharma drug companies who manufactured them. Those initial, industry funded NRT trials were over twice as likely to produce positive results as later independent ones. The earlier clinical

trials did not accurately reflect real world conditions and success rates were a vast over exaggeration. The drug company findings were misleading and the research woefully designed. Difficult to treat smokers were often excluded - such as people who also drank alcohol - even though this amounts to over 85 percent of smokers. Results were often published looking at people who had managed to quit for 6 months or less, rather than for a whole year. They also adopted the tactic of comparing NRT success rates to trial studies with unusually low success rate for willpower.

Even when those given NRT do manage to avoid smoking, full withdrawal is simply delayed until they eventually stop using NRT after a number of weeks. At this point nicotine withdrawal must finally be faced in any case, and according to anecdotal reports, it is as abrupt and difficult as if they had simply gone cold turkey in the first place. By comparison, those who choose to quit unaided from the word go are over any withdrawal after a few weeks and are already enjoying being non smokers.

Quit smoking is becoming increasingly medicalised - to the obvious benefit of pharmaceutical companies - hiding public awareness of the fact that the most successful way to quit is to do so unaided. In the UK The NHS spends an estimated £84million a year on drug assisted stop smoking programmes and has plans to spend even more.

Despite the consistent failure of quit smoking programmes, health authorities and quit smoking organisations regard it as somehow irresponsible or subversive to suggest anyone should attempt to quit without drugs. Quitting unassisted is seldom emphasised in advice to smokers. Smokers are be encouraged to do anything but go it alone when trying to quit - which is exactly how the vast majority of ex-smokers succeeded. This is a dangerous trend because it shifts the smokers locus of control away from believing they have the power to change their habits from within – to believing they need an outside force to change those habits.

The drug companies who manufacture NRT donate millions towards cancer and other health research which encourages governments to advise people to use their products. Not surprisingly lung associations, heart associations and cancer associations rarely, if ever, mention the merits of going cold turkey on their websites.

30 - Zyban (bupropion hydrochloride)

Zyban is supposed to reduce the severity of nicotine cravings and withdrawal symptoms. It was touted as a wonder cure drug when first launched, but an Australian survey in 2006 found that cold turkey success rates were twice as high as among those who were prescribed Zyban or NRT by their doctor (Doran et al 2006).

Zyban certainly comes with risks and side effects. It was famously linked to 35 deaths in the UK during its first year, including a number of young people who were previously healthy and had opted to take it in order to quit smoking. Formally used as an antidepressant, it suppresses the neurotransmitters dopamine and noradrenalin, the brain's "pleasure centres", which appear to be stimulated by nicotine.

UK Department of Health figures also showed that in its first year 3,457 Zyban users suffered a disturbing range of suspected side effects - from chest pains to fits, seizures and depression. In all, 7,600 reports of suspected adverse reactions were collected in the first two years after its approval. There have been many cases of patients suffering fits. The drug is known to cause epileptic seizures, causing it to be withdrawn from the market between 1986 and 1989.

31 - Champix (varenicline tartrate)

Champix is designed to help the smoker quit by blocking nicotine receptors in the brain and therefore making smoking pleasure impossible. Stopping nicotine from getting to the brain or blocking nicotine receptors doesn't help - for reasons which have already been discussed in the section on Champix in Chapter 22.

Never in the history of quit smoking products has any drug caused such a wide array of serious side effects, including death. Known to cause nightmarish hallucinatory type dreams, and suicidal thoughts.

Three studies pitted Champix against NRT (Aubin 2008, Tsukahara 2010 and Dhelaria 2012). In each, Champix failed to show statistical significance over NRT when looking at the percentage of quitters within each group who were still not smoking at 24 weeks.

The only reason the drug ever had any success is probably down to the placebo effect - in other words it is a drug that works simply because the person taking it simply believes it will.

32 - Planet of the Vapes

Generally speaking, the further anything is removed from nature, the more potentially deadly it becomes. The vape, or e-cigarette, is an artificial, electronic contrivance that is rapidly gaining in popularity all over the world. At this rate we will soon be living on The Planet of the Vapes!

Vapes are just as dangerous as conventional cigarettes and do not help you quit. A study at The University of California (Kalkhoran and Glantz, 2016) found that use of e-cigarettes in fact *lowered* a person's chance of successfully quitting cigarettes by 28%.

Vaping can do lasting and irreparable damage to cells, inducing increased DNA strand breaks and cell death. Vapes have also been linked to the incurable condition "popcorn lung" which results in scarring of tiny air sacs, so called because it first appeared in workers who inhaled artificial butter flavor in microwave popcorn processing facilities. A Harvard study by Allen et al (2016) found, 75 percent of flavoured e-cigarettes and their refill liquids were found to contain Diacetyl, a flavoring chemical linked to cases of severe respiratory disease. It's particularly disturbing because of the appeal fruity flavours such as "Cotton Candy, Fruit Squirts, and Cupcake" may have to young people.

Remember, whether you smoke or vape you are still a nicotine user. The problem isn't smoking - it's nicotine addiction. If you switch from smoking heroin to injecting it you have given nothing up. If you switch from smoking tobacco to vaping or using NRT you have given nothing up - you are still a nicotine user.

On the internet there are forums where smokers claim they have "quit smoking" because they have switched to e-cigarettes. That is ridiculous! If you are still unable to get through the day without inhaling the drug nicotine you are still a nicotine addict - regardless of how it is delivered.

Many former smokers, who have successfully overcome the hurdles of quitting have recently returned to nicotine use through taking up vaping. This is almost certainly because many of them feel deprived after quitting and are encouraged to return to what they regard as a useful drug by reassurances that taking it alone is safer than smoking it...or even harmless. This is a tragic situation for several reasons. Firstly, any ex - smoker returning to nicotine use will find themselves re-addicted to the drug, just as a easily as a returning heroine user is re-addicted to heroin if it is taken again. Consequently the returning nicotine user will begin to re-experience the constant lapses into withdrawal in between each dose, just as when they smoked cigarettes. Secondly vapes are no safer than cigarettes, and possibly more dangerous. Thirdly, as nicotine is by far the most poisonous ingredient in tobacco anyway, they will experience all the ongoing negative health consequences, as are outlined elsewhere in this book.

Furthermore, many vapers start consuming far more nicotine than before, without realising it, and become more addicted to the substance than ever, making it considerably harder to quit. It's so easy to start smoking the equivalent of 40 a day instead of the usual 20 for example. This

is because there is no longer the simple, traditional way of monitoring (and therefore limiting) the amount of nicotine consumed by counting the number of cigarettes you have smoked. Vape users talk of how they have managed to "quit", smoking and how relieved they are to be finally be free from the dangers of smoking. Hopefully after reading this book you will not suffer from the same delusion.

Hardly a week goes by without a tabloid article reporting a vape explosion. One of the first incidents was when a Florida man was almost killed when one blew up in his face, blowing out several of his teeth and part of his tongue. Red hot pieces of the fake cigarette were reported to have flown across the room. Ironically, the man was trying to quit smoking.

Nicotine is a deadly substance and almost certainly the most dangerous ingredient in tobacco smoke. Vaping causes cell mutations the same as tobacco smoke. Cells exposed to the e-cigarette vapour showed several forms of damage, including DNA strand breaks the same as those exposed to tobacco smoke. DNA damage is thought to be the root cause of cancer.

As with tobacco tar (of which nicotine is a component anyway) there is considerable evidence of a link between nicotine and cancer. A study recently carried out showed that when mice were given nicotine injections for two years - 78% of them developed cancer (Grando 2014).

A cancer study by Park et al (2014) studied bronchial cells in a culture medium and found that when the cells were exposed to e-cigarette vapour containing nicotine they showed similar gene mutations to cells exposed to tobacco smoke, and determined to be at risk of becoming cancerous.

When you vape you are inhaling propylene glycol (PG) - a household product often used as an ingredient in shampoos, pet foods, bubble bath, after shave, deodorants and baby wipes. "E-liquid," "or vape juice" is the key ingredients in e-cigarettes, and because of the nicotine content, it is a powerful neurotoxin. Even tiny amounts, if swallowed or absorbed through the skin, can cause vomiting and seizures and even be lethal. Vape juice comes in various flavours with names like "Apple Pie" or "Banana Creme." which can potentially attract small children. A sip of even highly diluted e-liquid can kill a child. Another dangerous chemical contained in about three quarters of all e-cigarettes is diacetyl, a flavouring that has been linked to lung disease.

A study looking a cell death by Yu et al (2016) concluded that E-cigarettes are no safer than regular smoking and can "cause cancer even when they're nicotine free." Toxins found in e-cigarettes trigger the same cell damage that causes cancer. One of the researchers, Professor Wang-Rodriquez said: "Based on the evidence to date, I believe they are no better than smoking regular cigarettes."

Many countries have now banned vaping. I predict that in about 10 years it will be shown, conclusively that vapes are considerably more deadly than cigarettes. I only hope this doesn't culminate in a kind of dreadful, science fiction type scenario a little further on into the 21st century. Imagine a nightmarish situation where people who have switched to e-cigarettes, or who have decided to return to "smoking" (believing there is now a safe alternative to tobacco) finally realise they now face far greater and more terrifying risks than ever before, coupled with having acquired a much deeper addiction to nicotine.

If you have moved to "The Planet of the Vapes" or are thinking of going there - think again! Don't believe the clever advertising hype that makes out that electronic cigarettes are a smart, modern, safe, sexy, healthier, or guilt free alternative to smoking. Do yourself a favour and keep well away from them. If you already have a vape throw it in the bin right now!

33 - A Spliff Smoker is a Cigarette Smoker

A spliff or a joint is really a kind of cigarette with a small addiction of cannabis, which means that a spliff smoker is basically just another kind of nicotine user. The main content of a joint is usually, or though not always, tobacco. In reality it is a large, rolled cigarette with a small addition of cannabis or grass. Some people insist that a spliff is a spliff and not basically cigarette with something added. That's like saying a larger and lime is not basically a larger.

Whereas nicotine is a stimulant drug, cannabis acts as a sedative and mood enhancer right from the first dose. Although it is a genuine sedative, people who are habitually drugging themselves with it in large doses are really only half alive. The negative side effects are legendary - personality changes, false confidence, overbearing behaviour, minor delusions, paranoia, depression, lethargy and anti social behaviour. An overdose can be terrifying, causing temporary psychosis, depersonalisation and derealisation, reminiscent of a bad LSD trip.

Cannabis is a very mild drug compared to nicotine and when taken alone, does not appear to be physically addictive. The belief amongst cannabis users that they are hooked on cannabis alone, stems from ignorance about the addictive nature of nicotine, which is almost always a component of a spliff. They are indeed hooked, but hooked on the highly addictive nicotine in the tobacco rather than to the cannabis. This means that once you have quit cigarettes or vapes, you cannot smoke a joint, as even taking a puff will almost certainly re-addict you to nicotine.

At the very least you will go into nicotine withdrawal over the next few days without realise what it is. For example, you will feel down, irritable and unsettled - much like occasional smokers do in the days that follow their occasional cigarettes.

Whereas nicotine is a deadly poison, cannabis it is no more poisonous than say carrots or peas. It also has many medicinal properties. It cannot harm the body physically in any dose, unless smoked, but then again, almost every natural substance on the planet becomes potentially harmful once it is smoked. This is because once you burn any organic substance you produce chemicals, such as nitrosamines, that can damage DNA and this can affect cell growth and cause cancer.

34 - Lennox Johnston and Allen Carr

The notion that nicotine is pointless and as a recreational drug was first put forward in the 1940s by the Scottish physician Lennox Johnston. It was then broadcast more widely by the quit smoking guru Allen Carr in 1983, but there were shortcomings in the way both of them put forward their arguments. Large chunks of the complicated jigsaw were still missing, and I believe this is why the truth about nicotine failed to become generally understood or accepted by the public, health organisations, and scientific community alike. Nearly a century after Johnston, scientific research into smoking still makes the assumption that nicotine has the ability to act as a sedative.

Lennox Johnston

As mentioned in the chapter on addiction, Johnston, was the first person ever to carry out research into the addictive nature of nicotine. In the 1940s he gave 35 of his patients nicotine injections and found he could wean them off smoking to such an extent that the injections were generally preferred to smoking. Once the injections ceased, cravings quickly arose, reminiscent of those experienced by heroin or cocaine addicts. He found that one milligram of injected nicotine was roughly the equivalent of smoking one cigarette. In a letter to the Lancet (1942) he concluded that "smoking tobacco is essentially a means of administering nicotine, just as smoking opium is a means of administering morphine."

Johnston them went on to claim:

"No smoker derives positive pleasure and benefit from tobacco. The bliss of headache or toothache relieved is analogous to that of craving for tobacco appeased."

This revolutionary view - that nicotine was an addictive drug that had no recreational value - was all but completely ignored by The British Medical Association. This is hardly surprising as they already viewed him as an eccentric crank because of his constant campaigning against smoking on health grounds.

Johnston also put other recreational drugs, such as cocaine in the same useless bracket as nicotine, based on his own experience with the drug when he was unable to derive any pleasure until he had taken several doses. He came to the conclusion:

"The pleasure arising from of drugs of addiction arises mainly from the appeasement of craving once such craving has been acquired" (Lancet 1952)

Here I disagree with Johnston. Heroin and cocaine users say the complete opposite - that the first ever dose is especially pleasurable and intense, especially in the case of heroin. Smokers (nicotine users) on the other hand invariably report no drug pleasure from first time use. Therefore I believe that nicotine is unique in being the only recreational drug on the planet that is incapable of providing any positive pleasure. In other words it is the only drug of addiction where all the pleasure arises from appeasement of craving.

Lennox continued to demand the BMA publish his research linking smoking to lung cancer and other diseases, the first person ever to do so, but the BMA consistently refused to fund his research or publish any of his papers, much to Johnston's anger and frustration. Most of the BMA were smokers themselves. Johnston had good reason to be angry - there is no doubt that hundreds of thousands of lives would have been saved if the BMA had taken action earlier. Their dogged refusal to listen to Johnston for some *thirty years* was not because they lacked intelligence or goodwill, it was because turning against smoking, or even admitting that nicotine was an addictive drug, required a massive paradigm change.

A similar paradigm change is required now. Doctors and researchers need to drop the outdated view that smoking is the primary problem - and see it as nicotine use. Research into quitting should be aimed primarily at nicotine use. If people switch from smoking to vaping they are still nicotine users. If people switch from smoking to nicotine patches or gum they are still nicotine users. Sometimes I feel as frustrated as Johnston did!

Alan Carr

In 1983, the well known quit smoking guru, Allen Carr was one of the first authors to claim that smoking was a useless trap and that quitting involved no sacrifice. Many of the views he expresses in his "Easy way to Stop Smoking" book are diametrically opposite to my own, but the book was a phenomenal success and doubtless saved countless lives. Despite this, it now sounds fairly dated and I believe has a number of flaws which can actually hinder people from stopping. Also, it is mostly from the perspective of the very heavy smoker, which is quite natural as he was one himself.

For the benefit of anyone who has failed to quit after reading Allen Carr, I have itemised how his views differ fundamentally to my own:

1. Pleasure denial

In Allen Carr's *Easyway*, the claim is repeatedly made that there is no pleasure in smoking - which is very confusing to smokers. *Quit Smoking in Style* doesn't do this. To tell a smoker they are experiencing no pleasure is untrue - it amounts to telling them to deny their own experience or senses. Of course there is a pleasure in coming out of drug withdrawal, regardless as to whether it is withdrawal from a drug capable of giving pleasure such as alcohol or opium, or a drug incapable of doing so, such as nicotine or Paracetamol. *Quit Smoking in Style* makes it clear there *is* a pleasure but goes to great length to explain why the pleasure is useless and pointless.

As stressed many times in *Quit Smoking in Style* - the pleasure of smoking is of course real, but paradoxically it isn't coming from the drug itself. It is the brain rewarding you for replenishing the drug, which is something totally different. Nicotine is a stimulant that can't relax you, which is why, ironically, the drug is totally useless.

2. Withdrawal denial

Carr believed that once the message (that nicotine is pointless) is understood withdrawal is avoided.

Quit Smoking in Style doesn't make this claim. It doesn't make smokers think they shouldn't be experiencing withdrawal if they have fully understood the message. It is quite true that some lucky people experience no withdrawal at all, but even people who fully comprehend why nicotine is useless can still get withdrawal, because the desire for an addictive drug arises subconsciously from the autonomic nervous system, rather like the desire for food and water. In other words it's something you can't switch off through an act of will, unless somehow you can override a subconscious process, which is only possible through something like hypnosis. Regardless of its severity, withdrawal is so much more bearable once you realise you are making no sacrifice by giving up nicotine.

3. There is no Nicotine Monster

Carr demonised the part of the mind or body that craves nicotine calling it the "Nicotine Monster." There is no "Nicotine Monster". The brain is actually trying to help you by producing nicotine cravings.

There is need to demonise your cravings when you quit. There is no metaphorical monster to do battle with. Ironically, it would appear that the automatic part of the brain is trying to help you by creating the desire to smoke. That desire is simply the brain's way of ensuring that nicotine levels are topped up, as if the substance was essential to the body, rather like the way it makes you thirsty when your body is running low on water.

Believing there is a negative force within you to do battle against is unhelpful. It's a bit like inferring that a crying baby is deliberately creating trouble, or giving it a nickname like "noise devil" rather than understanding that it's crying out of instinct. If cravings occur, they are not being created by an act of will, they are arising automatically from the subconscious mind. Although cravings may be a nuisance if they occur, try and embrace the unconscious part of your mind or body that produces that niggle or craving for a cigarette. Do not think of it as a nicotine monster you must overpower, starve, or kill. Treat it with understanding and love, rather than see it as an enemy. The subconscious mind is just a machine or computer with the wrong programming. It doesn't realise that nicotine is useless and unnecessary. If it produces a craving for nicotine it is only trying to help.

4. The dangers of smoking

Carr repeatedly states that informing smokers of the dangers of smoking is unhelpful and will not help them quit.

"Quit Smoking In Style" takes the opposite view. *Part Two* is all about the dangers of smoking. I believe that knowing as much as possible about the risks of smoking is helpful to quitting, especially when it comes to reducing the numbers of smokers who return to smoking after a period of being a successful non smoker. Smoking is a dangerous trap and the more wary you are of the dangers the more likely you are to escape and the less likely you are to return. In addition, I believe the history of smoking is also important. Learning how we came to smoke in the first place, how unnatural the modern practice of smoking is, with its chemical treatment and additives, is very eye opening and motivational.

5. Willpower

Carr led smokers to believe that willpower is unnecessary in order to quit so long as the smoker understands the message that taking nicotine is pointless. This ties in with his belief there should be no withdrawal - for the same reason.

I have massive respect for Carr, but to be honest saying you won't need willpower is a bit of an outlandish claim - reminiscent of the kind of thing you find in the more sensation seeking self help books. Telling smokers they won't need willpower sets up unrealistic expectations and consequent disappointment for those who find that they certainly do need it, which can lead to losing faith in the notion that no sacrifice is being made from a drug point of view. Prior to writing the book he had visited a hypnotherapist who very likely hypnotised him to have no desire to smoke, and that he would experience no withdrawal symptoms - which could easily explain why he himself required no willpower on quitting, especially if he was a good hypnotic subject.

All his conclusions about smoking were based on his own subjective experience. Previously he had only ever worked as an accountant and as far as I know had no experience of helping anyone quit smoking.

In contrast I wrote Quit Smoking in Style on the back of twenty years helping smokers quit at the sharp end, and in my experience those who are aware that smoking has no benefit still need willpower, although it is likely to be considerably less.

6. Vaping

"Quit Smoking in Style" is addressed to *nicotine users* rather than just to just to smokers. Smokers are basically just a subset of nicotine users, albeit the largest one. The book is more focused on nicotine addiction rather than seeing it as just smoking addiction. This is important

in the Twenty First Century as many smokers turn to vaping as an alternative to smoking. The basic problem isn't smoking, it's nicotine addiction.

7. Cannabis

A spliff is actually a type of cigarette. The main difference is that it has a small amount of cannabis (marijuana or "grass") added in one form or another. Carr doesn't tackle the issue of spliff smoking (also known as smoking a joint or dope) but it is so widespread, especially amongst young smokers, that understanding how it is linked to tobacco and nicotine addiction is crucial. If you smoke spliffs you are also a tobacco smoker and therefore a nicotine user (the only exception being if you smoke pure grass). You are almost certainly addicted to the nicotine rather than the cannabis.

8. Scientific angle

In the age of the internet anyone can quickly discover that conventional scientific wisdom assumes that, regardless of any health risks, nicotine can

148

provide positive benefit to the user. "Quit Smoking in Style" therefore takes a much more scientific look at nicotine addiction than Carr's "Easyway".

When people learn from online sources that the brain produces pleasure neurotransmitters such as dopamine during smoking, they challenge the notion that nicotine is a useless drug. Quit Smoking in Style explains that these neurotransmitters are only released to reward the addict for replenishing nicotine, pointing out that the brain also releases reward neurotransmitters when we replenish non drug substances such as water.

Carr's book stops short of attempting to provide a scientific explanation as to why taking nicotine is pointless. There is also no research information to back up any of the statistics quoted - you just have to accept his word for things.

35 - Vested interests of Tobacco Companies, Big Pharma and Governments

Statistically speaking, nicotine is by far and away the world's most dangerous drug, yet it is completely legal to be a dealer or supplier.

William Morris, the world's tobacco company, make over four billion dollars profit a year (2005). A third of the world's adult population now smoke. Use is rising in the developing world. There are more Chinese smokers (300 million) than there are citizens of the United States.

As mentioned earlier, no tobacco company boss wants their loved ones to smoke. In fact tobacco companies are now spending millions trying to develop a safe cigarette, or at least a safer cigarette one. This follows increasing legislation against smoking which is a real threat to cigarette sales.

It's not just tobacco companies that have a vested interest in people continuing to smoke or vape - the pharmaceutical companies do to, because they make billions out of selling nicotine products such as patches, gum and various other drugs that independent studies consistently show do not help people quit. Big Pharma make generous donations to health charities and in return receive huge government subsidies and research funds for their drugs. Critics of this cosy arrangement say it encourages health authorities to recommend people take NRT and other drugs, even though statistically, quitting unaided has a far better success rate. A cynical view might be - if every smoker were to quit, the demand for such drugs would cease, so you could argue the fact that they do not work is good for business!

Governments themselves make fortunes out of smokers through tax. They have never made being a nicotine dealer or supplier a criminal offence because historically so many of their members, and the public, have been nicotine users themselves. In the UK, nearly 90% of the price of a packet of cigarettes is tax earning the government roughly **£12 billion a year** in tobacco revenue.

This funds roughly 10% of the entire annual NHS budget. The annual burden to the NHS of treating smoking related diseases is estimated to be about **£2 billion** (Local costs of smoking, 2015 Action on Smoking and Health). New research smoking costs NHS 5 billion a year.

Needless to say, it would be a lot more cost effective if they handed out copies of this book instead!

Smoking bans

The culture of shame surrounding smoking is on the increase. Smokers are increasingly being marginalised by the introduction of smoking bans in public places. Australia has introduced mandatory plain packaging for tobacco products and is steadily increasing tax on cigarettes each year, in an attempt to reduce the number of smokers. UK is soon to introduce a similar plain packaging law. In developed countries, the majority of people who smoke are now at the bottom end of the socio-economic scale and there is no real evidence that increasing taxes causes any reduction in smoking. All taxes and bans do is cause resentment and unnecessary hardship to smokers and their families. These days it's the poor who are most likely to smoke and the culture of shame is as divisive as it is counter productive. Smokers resent the heavy hand of the law, and decreasing personal liberty can have the opposite effect of encouraging people to quit. As happened with alcohol prohibition, a total ban would simply drive smoking underground, where it would resurface with cult status. It would doubtless cause a new wave of drug related crime - the scale of which the world has never previously known, plus there would be no controls on what goes into tobacco.

Cannabis had been illegal in many countries for decades - but has that ever stopped anyone or discouraged young people from taking up the drug? The leaders and presidents of many countries have now owned up to having smoked weed. All banning does is make a drug go underground and cause divisions within society.

Part Four
How to Quit Smoking in Style

"Giving up smoking is the easiest thing in the world. I know because I've done it thousands of times!"
- Mark Twain

36 - Using the Power of the Mind

The aim of his book has been to summon and release the power of your mind through telling you the surprising truth about smoking. This section contains guidance, but there is no separate list of instructions as to how to quit because every word in this book is part of that instruction. The information is designed to get you to harness and magnify the power of your mind, turning it into an unstoppable force, making it much, much easier for you to stop!

As I said at the start of this book, quitting smoking is like ending a useless relationship - you just walk away completely and permanently. Do people need to memorise a complex list of instructions in order to end a relationship? No.

Hopefully, what you have learned so far has already had a profound effect over the way you think and feel about smoking. This, in turn should have a massive effect on the amount, if any, of craving or withdrawal you experience when you quit. Some withdrawal is physical, but the mind and body is actually just one continuum and what happens in the mind has an ongoing effect on what happens to the body.

Be reassured that most smokers eventually manage to quit. In The UK and USA there are now more ex-smokers than smokers! This means that YOU can do it too. How did they do it? Roughly 90% of them did it through the power of the mind - in other words through willpower. The way to learn how to do anything well is to copy from the people who do it the best, whether it's flying aircraft, brain surgery, going to the Moon or quit smoking, and statistically the most effective way of stopping smoking is just stopping unaided. Stopping without drugs or mentoring, i.e. willpower or cold turkey.

Willpower is not only the best way, it's the easiest way. No looking back, no cutting down, no stopping and starting, no drugs, no mentors, no weekly lectures. No need for a plan. Once you quit there's only one cigarette or vape you have to avoid the rest of your life - the first one.

Nicotine gum, patches and other quit smoking drugs have been heavily promoted for over twenty years, yet they have only worked for a fraction of those who have tried them - and even that success was probably down to the placebo effect. This means that statistically, willpower is by far the best way of stopping smoking.

Drug companies have a vested interest in promoting the idea that smokers are foolish to try quitting on their own and need professional help or drugs, yet despite the almost universal availability of these drugs over the past 20 years, quitting unaided has remained the most common way that people have quit successfully.

37 - The Mindset of the Person who Quits Easily

The mindset of the person who quits easily and with minimal unpleasantness is simply that of unshakable determination. Only when there is no question of ever smoking or vaping again - regardless of what happens - does the brain let you relax in situations where you used to smoke.

Once you are aware that by quitting you are giving up absolutely nothing (from a drug point of view) it is much easier to obtain that mindset, compared to someone who believes that they are making a sacrifice for the sake of their health.

In order to quit successfully you do not need to read and memorise a complicated set of instructions - you simply need to have that mindset. Everything you have read so far in this book has been about giving you that mindset.

Remember - You became addicted to a drug that cannot relax you. A drug that has never relaxed or given pleasure to any human being, a bit like becoming hooked on something like Paracetamol or Trap-eze. You were a slave to a useless drug, a slave to the world's most useless recreational drug.

Here is a little summary of what you now know:

Although dangerous, smoking appears to provide a crutch and a boost that non smokers do not get. The suggestion that smoking is useless from a drug point of view goes against the grain of everything we have assumed about cigarettes since we were small children watching adults smoke. It appears at odds with commonsense and even our own experience as we draw in smoke or nicotine vapour. Almost everyone assumes that nicotine has a benefit from a drug point of view - smokers, ex. smokers and non smokers alike, by scientists, doctors and even quit smoking organisation.

*The pleasurable effects **are not in doubt** - but that is not why the drug is useless. The reason nicotine is useless is that one hundred percent of those pleasurable effects are caused by the elimination of the drug withdrawal symptoms, which accumulate between each cigarette or dose of nicotine. In other words, they are the pleasurable sensation of returning to the normal state - which non smokers experience all the time - the state of being free from nicotine withdrawal symptoms.*

It's much easier to give something up once you know it is totally useless. Whether it is a friendship, a relationship, a job, a way of life or a drug. Once you've completely made up your mind for sure about something, there's nothing to think about or discuss.

38 - How to actually quit

As soon as you have read enough of the book to posses the mindset described above you are ready.

Simply pick a day and time to stop. Have your last cigarette or vape, then throw away all cigarettes, lighters, tobacco, vapes, gum, patches, ash trays - everything - and quit.

If you have understood why cigarettes are absolutely useless at relaxing you, you will find the withdrawal much more mild or even nonexistent because you will realise you are making no sacrifice. Remember - only when there is 'no question' of ever touching another cigarette the rest of your life does the calm ever really come.

If you find it difficult to recall why nicotine is useless in a factual, logical way just remember one of the crazy stories - like the Rhino Story, The Stappie Story, The Paracetamol Story, or The Trap-Eze Story. Everything you need to know and remember about the pointlessness of smoking or vaping is in those stories.

To summarise - in order to minimise or eliminate withdrawal symptoms you must be completely sure of two things:

1. That nicotine has absolutely no benefit to any human being, 2. That you will never, ever smoke or take nicotine in any shape or form for the rest of your life.

Once you are genuinely sure of those two things, something deep down in the mind will change. Something lets go at a very profound level which affects all of the mind and the body. You may notice a feeling of elation and freedom. This can only happen once you resolve you will never smoke again whatever happens.

39 - Ritual and visualisation

This is optional, but the following visualisation will help communicate the fact you are quitting to the subconscious part of your mind, that otherwise might be completely unaware you are quitting. Ritual and visualisation are both very powerful ways of getting the unconscious, automatic processes of the mind and body to understand that a major change is happening in your life and to react in accordance with your will.

Just before you quit, find a time and place when you can maybe sit and pause for a while. Preferably somewhere warm and comfortable. Switch off your phone. Relax, close your eyes and become aware of all of the sounds going on around you. Do not block any sound. Allow the everyday world to continue without you for a while. Take in a deep breath or two and exhale. Then visualise yourself quitting with incredible power, determination and confidence, surprising anyone who knows you. It does not matter how clearly you see the visualisation. Imagine yourself as one of those lucky people who experiences absolutely no withdrawal symptoms at all, going right through a typical day not wanting to smoke or vape.

Open your eyes at any time if you need to refresh your mind about any aspect of the visualisation, otherwise keep them closed.

Imagine looking around yourself as a non smoker, proud to be a non smoker, refusing cigarettes without apology or hesitation. Imagine people you used to smoke with holding aloft a cigarette or vape in between puffs. As you do this recall the Strappie Story, and using your imagination change the cigarette or vape they are holding into one of the tight Strappies. There is nothing to envy. Being a smoker or vaper is as pointless as being a Strappie wearer. See yourself being amused that they are unwittingly just in a pointless trap. Imagine yourself having no desire to smoke and being relieved to be free of a completely useless and pointless drug, becoming healthier, stronger, fitter with every day. Imagine becoming calmer in every situation in life and better able to handle stress - which is possibly the greatest benefit of all.

Imagine the days going by as a successful non smoker, see yourself at home, at work, after food, maybe out having a drink or coffee as a successful non smoker. On all of those occasions imagine that for some reason you have absolutely no desire to smoke or vape whatsoever.

Imagine a little child who has lost one of its parents to smoking weeping alone. You go up to the child, you bob down in front of it and tear up your last cigarettes. You then stand up in front of the child, proud to be a non smoker and the child looks up at you, managing a faint but brave smile. You have chosen life, health, strength, beauty and above all...freedom from the world's most completely and utterly useless drug, nicotine.

Solemnly swear to yourself you will never touch a cigarette or nicotine in any shape or form ever again. Inform the very deepest most powerful parts of your mind or body that all along nicotine was a useless stimulant drug and that you will never smoke or use nicotine the rest of your life. Then slowly open your eyes as a non smoker, celebrate as you throw away the cigarettes, tobacco or vapes and then forget all about smoking or vaping. If cigarettes or vapes every come into your mind again just celebrate the fact you are now utterly free from a completely useless and pointless drug and forget about it again. Just carry on with your life. You are now free! You are now a non smoker!

40 - Hypnotherapy

If you want to go a stage further than visualisation you can always seek the professional help of a hypnotherapist.

As a hypnotherapist for over 20 years I am aware of the tremendous role the subconscious mind plays not only in addiction, and producing the desire to smoke, but also in helping people quit. Hypnotherapy is easily the most effective way of quitting on the planet. I have personally conducted thousands of successful quit smoking sessions. All of them using the message in this book coupled with a hypnosis session.

I recommend anyone quitting smoking, or vaping - not just those who are struggling - to strongly consider using hypnotherapy in conjunction with this book. Amongst other things hypnosis utilises the power of suggestion to reduce or remove the desire to smoke, builds up motivation, determination and willpower, and gets the smoker to visualise the future as a successful non smoker. The power of the subconscious (unconscious) mind is phenomenal. Hypnotherapy can communicate with that power and direct it so that it works on your behalf rather than against you - like reprogramming a computer. I believe that one day hypnosis, in conjunction with visualisation, will be used routinely by everyone who wishes to make positive changes in their life.

I believe that many smokers who read Allen Carr's "Easyway to Quit Smoking" book, which was first published in 1983, were put off hypnotherapy because he claimed it did not work for him. Although not against hypnotherapy, Carr famously visited a hypnotherapist just before he quit and says he did it "in spite of him, not because of him."

According to Carr, despite years of struggling with smoking, it was soon after this visit that he received the epiphany that inspired him to write his book. He gives no credit to the hypnotherapist for quitting, but in my profession this is not uncommon. Many people expect to lose consciousness during hypnosis. When this does not happen, they claim, as Carr did, that they were not hypnotised. They do not realise that rather than being a form of controlling people, hypnosis is an empowerment. It is designed to release the individual's own power.

Carr lit up immediately after the session but then quit with spectacular ease and no withdrawal very soon afterwards. He did eventually admit that he was able to quit because the hypnotherapist had told him smoking was "just nicotine addiction." Apparently, this revelation was also one of the main things that inspired him to write his book!

Many good hypnotic subjects experience post hypnotic amnesia - they cannot recall what was said to them during hypnosis - and therefore give the hypnotist no credit for any sudden new belief, realisation or breakthrough. This is by no means untypical. Virtually all hypnotherapists tell clients that smoking is pointless when they are in a trance. They are professionals who have a vested interest in success. Since the 1960s, many have specialised in quit smoking, they are highly trained, well read and knowledgeable about addictions of all kinds. This is very likely how Carr finally came to learn of the views of Lennox Johnston. On the other hand, he may coincidentally have worked it all out for himself independently - immediately after the session. We shall never know.

Carr's reluctance to recommend any smoker to visit a mainstream hypnotherapist was no doubt partly due to the fact that hypnotherapy was the main competitor for his own, highly lucrative quit smoking seminar business. Despite saying it didn't work for him, he went on to use hypnotherapy as an integral part of those seminars! If he didn't believe in it - why did he incorporate it into those sessions?

41 - Celebrate!

As you quit... celebrate! It means that by quitting you are giving nothing up. You have been a slave to a completely useless drug and quitting involves no sacrifice whatsoever. You are escaping from the worst trap of your life. Sometimes escaping from a trap involves pain - other times there is none - but either way it is a time to celebrate!

Every single cigarette you ever smoked was useless from a drug point of view. Everyone was pointless. You took a risk and damaged your body for nothing. Everyone who has ever smoked was also hooked on a useless drug - Winston Churchill, King George 6th, Einstein, John Lennon, Kate Moss, and...yes...you! All the countless millions who smoked through history, all fell prey to this trap.

42 - Unshakeable Determination

My dad quit smoking with amazing ease! I'm not one of those people who idolises their father. Many people regarded him as a bit of a loser, and he had little respect from within his own family. He never made much money or held down a job for long, he always seemed to go against the grain of life in general. Never the less, he was very much his own person. He bought a massive house, had four children, was the life and soul of parties, and always dressed in style. In fact he more or less did everything in style. When he wanted to he could make just about anything fun, more often than not going against the grain of convention in a way I learned to admire. He was outspoken and by comparison, made my friends parents look like sheep.

He was also a heavy smoker.

One day, when I was about nine or ten, he announced to the family he had quit. My brother and I exchanged knowing glances, both convinced he would weaken, so when he came home from work that evening we taunted him as he ate his dinner, teasing him about quitting, trying to tempt him and weaken his resolve, saying how a cigarette would make him feel much better, going on about how much he must be dying for one. We went on like this, either side of him for some time but my dad seemed to totally ignore us. Eventually, he put down his knife and fork and looked at us both.

"Boys" he said. "You don't seem to understand. There's no question of me having another cigarette the rest of my life"

With that he just picked up his newspaper and became engrossed in it. I mean completely engrossed. I looked across the table at my brother, both of us a bit shocked and disappointed that our attempts to tempt him had failed. At that moment both of us knew for certain that my dad would never ever smoke again. He didn't.

How did he do it?

Was it strength? Was it determination? Was it toughness? Was it wisdom? Was it Willpower?

It was *unshakeable determination.*

By ruling it out totally and for good, he quit smoking in style. He chucked away his last cigarettes and never once looked back. By doing this he appeared to sidestep withdrawal completely. I learned a lot about my dad that day, he was obviously a lot stronger or wiser than I had realised. I also learnt a lot about drug withdrawal. Years later, that incident enabled me to help thousands of other people quit. To quit in style like my dad.

Once you've quit, don't even think about going back. Don't toy with the idea of going back if things get particularly rough. People who make a song and dance about quitting are most likely to fail - and that's definitely not quitting in style!

You see, only when there is no question of ever smoking again does the calm come. Only when every single cell in your brain knows that nicotine will never again enter your body in any shape or form does it let you relax. This is why even very heavy smokers often report experiencing no craving for a cigarette on long haul plane flights. It's because they know there is no question of smoking for the duration of the flight. This just goes to show how much power the mind has over the amount of withdrawal we experience. if it can be done for the duration of a day long flight it can be done indefinitely! We have so much latent power within our minds, so much more than most people even begin to realise, but only when you make up your mind that there is no question of ever touching a cigarette or nicotine in any shape or form ever again does this work. The brain responds to unshakable determination like nothing else. This is why it's so important to quit smoking in style.

The softly, softly taking NRT for example is the complete opposite of this, which is why it makes quitting so much more miserable and pathetic. It is also why it fails 95% of the time. It's given out by people who underestimate the power of the mind and who don't have the faintest idea how about how the mind works. NRT is an example of the current day mentality, fuelled by drug company pressure, of handing out pharmaceuticals like candy because they make out they are the solution to everything.

43 - How you feel and look once you quit

The idea that you have to wait weeks, months or even years before you truly benefit from being a non smoker is just another myth.

One of the first things you will notice, a day or so after quitting, is a huge rise in energy levels. You will no longer feel tired and lethargic as often as you did. You do not have to wait until your lungs clear of tar for this to happen. This sudden rise in energy is due to the fact that the body no longer has the ongoing task of excreting the deadly poisons of smoking - especially nicotine. Some smokers find this new energy a little agitating or irritating, mainly because they are unaccustomed to it and fail to take advantage of it. They mistake it for a withdrawal symptom, which technically it is, but it should be regarded as a *positive* withdrawal symptom. Smokers who believe they are sacrificing a helpful drug when they quit frequently feel deprived and irritable in any case, and the excess energy typically compounds the situation. This is why some smokers resort to pacing up and down after they have quit. It can actually make you feel better because it uses up the new, surplus energy!

Quitting smoking is like recovering from a long term, low grade illness or infection. Energy levels rise quickly after many illnesses because toxin levels in the blood fall dramatically. If you were ever forced to remain in bed after recovering from an illness as a child, you will know what I am talking about. Imagine a child forced to remain in bed because it's parents do not realise it has fully recovered from an illness. At the height of the bug the child is stationary and lethargic because it's body was full of toxins, but now the poisons have gone the child experiences a massive surge in energy. It wants to get up, it can hear other children playing outside and longs to join them. Instead, it is forced to remain in bed a further two days. It tosses and turns in the bed, in an attempt to be free of the surplus energy. It has the most agitating two days of its life.

Smokers can find themselves in a similar situation when they quit. Toxins leave the body quickly, energy levels rise but many smokers do not use up all this surplus energy, so like the child who is forced to say in bed, agitation quickly follows. Typically, smokers avoid socialising when they quit, they cut down on all kinds of activities, they stop going out. They remain still while the energy levels rise. The best way to handle this surplus energy when you quit is to become more active, and enjoy moving around more. Welcome that energy! On top of that, you'll find you get far less easily fatigued than usual do everyday things such as chores.

Remember, you are simply experiencing the return of your own, natural energy levels, which you are unaccustomed to. Your body is urging you to get up, move around and use the new surplus energy.

Over the first few days and weeks you will also notice a steady increase in stamina, strength, fitness, and overall physical power. As the lungs continue to clear, aerobic capacity will also increase. You will notice more sparkle, more zing, more get up and go. Nothing will seem to be quite such an effort.

Unnatural aging of the skin will cease, and you will soon notice how much healthier your skin is becoming. There will be more glow and colour and you will almost certainly start looking a little younger. The improvement in the appearance of your skin will give you a reassuring indication as to how hidden damage within the organs and every part of the body is now being repaired. Every organ in your body will work more efficiently. Your immune system will become stronger and more efficient. Your circulation will improve and any coldness in the hands or feet, directly caused by smoking, will begin to disappear.

You will breathe more easily as your lungs start to repair. Your libido and sexual stamina will improve, especially if you were a heavy smoker. Your hair and clothes will no longer smell like a smoky dustbin. Your teeth, mouth and breath will be fresher and cleaner. Your sense of smell will improve and your taste buds will grow back to life!

None of these physical benefits however, even begins to compare to the greatest advantage of being a non smoker, which is that you become CALMER. You will find it easier to handle every situation in your life. This is partly because you are no longer putting a useless stimulant drug into your body, meaning your blood pressure will quickly return to normal, and also because you will no longer be descending into withdrawal between every cigarette or vape. The more you understand that by quitting you are making no sacrifice from a drug point of view, the quicker and the deeper the calm will be. You will experience a far deeper foundation of calm beneath every moment of your life, whether you are relaxing, working, physically active, alert or excited. There will be a deeper calm beneath everything you do.

When you wake up every day you have more energy, more vitality. You can run faster, do everything better! It means you will be able to enjoy every aspect of your life a little more, breathing nothing but beautiful, clear air into your body!

You will become richer. At £9 a packet in the UK, the average 20 a day smoker now spends roughly £60 a week on smoking. This works out at about £3000 per year, so why not reward yourself with a nice treat or exotic holiday with the money you will save by quitting? You deserve it!

44 - Gain more control over your weight

Many ex - smokers actually *lose* weight when they quit! This is because exercise no longer feels like an unpleasant chore, and the rapid return of energy, fitness, stamina and muscle power when you quit is legendary. Top athletes and sports people rarely smoke, not just because it compromises lung function but also because it poisons and slows down the body generally. Feelings of tiredness and lethargy no longer dampen your motivation to exercise once you have quit, and you too can lose weight - if that is your goal.

There is no need to substitute chocolate, confectionery, food, alcohol or anything else for those useless cigarettes or vapes you have dumped into your past. As mentioned earlier, when you quit your taste buds will grow back. They will come alive for healthier, fresher foods full of minerals, nutrients and vitamins that you will now be able to taste. Foods like salads and vegetables transform and become delicious, succulent and appertising because you can now experience their subtle flavours. Lettuce, for example, no longer tastes like green blotting paper! You will no longer be forced to rely on strong flavoured, salty, fatty, unhealthy food in order to taste anything properly. This means that potentially you will have far more control over what you eat and drink, and therefore over your weight. In fact, as a non smoker you will have more control over every aspect of your life!

It's true that nicotine suppresses the appetite, but it does so because it is one of the world's deadliest poisons. All deadly poisons spoil the appetite if taken in small doses. Arsenic, for example, if consumed in tiny amounts everyday will cause anyone to gradually lose weight without killing them - but who in their right mind would do this? Who, on earth would deliberately put a lethal poison into their body in order to control their weight?

Arsenic was famously used by persecuted Victorian women as a means of slowly murdering their husbands by adding the white powder to food. It was easy to achieve this because the damage gradually being caused was virtually impossible to detect. Likewise, if you smoke or vape in order to suppress your appetite you are slowly and progressively damaging your body at such a slow rate the damage may not be noticeable, and yet you are slowly killing yourself. In fact, ounce per ounce, nicotine is more toxic to the human body than arsenic.

Underweight or skinny people who may have struggled for years to gain weight will find that their muscle mass starts to increase as soon as they have quit smoking and that exercise has a far more positive effect on weight gain.

45 - Cravings...be tough but kind

S hould any cravings to smoke ever occur again do not demonise those cravings, it is simply the brain's automatic programming trying to get you to top up with a substance it genuinely believes is essential for the human body, rather like it calls for food, water and air when those levels get low. The brain simply couldn't care less whether nicotine is a drug or not. It doesn't care whether the drug stimulates you, relaxes you or takes you as high as a kite! It's just mistakenly programmed to believe that nicotine is essential for you. It's as if the brain comes to regard nicotine as some kind of essential vitamin, compound or fatty acid that is vital for your health or even survival! The brain may be confusing nicotine with acetylcholine, an essential neurotransmitter. Nicotine locks to the same sensors in the brain as acetylcholine. When this happens, the whole system then gets confused, and the brain starts to call for more and more nicotine.

It is not a situation where your mind is weakening, and calling out for a substance it knows brings you pleasure, it is more like a disc error in the computer part of your brain that is programmed to make sure you top up with essential substances!

So instead of demonising or resenting any desire or craving which arises automatically, be kind yet firm with those annoying pangs, in much the same way you would ignore a child who persistently and unreasonably has tantrums. In both cases here's no need to feel or show anger or resentment, you simply make it clear there is no way you are giving in, you do the best you can muster to ignore all the fuss, and simply get on with ordinary, everyday life.

Some people routinely give in to unreasonable children who have tantrums - and some people give in to the desire to smoke. In both cases, it's not because those people are weak or stupid. Far from it, they are often very tough, powerful and intelligent people...it's just that they are never really convinced that completely ruling out giving in is the right answer. It is.

Why give in to a faulty programming? As long as you ignore any desire to smoke, over time the brain (or mind/body continuum if you like) realises that nicotine is not essential after all, normal programming is resumed, at which point all desire and craving for nicotine ceases. The corrupted disc then remains dormant in the brain, but if at any time in the future nicotine re-enters the body the disc is immediately reactivated and calls for the same amount of nicotine as before.

46 - Cutting down is a myth

Nobody successfully cuts down. The only way to quit successfully is to abruptly cut out nicotine totally and forever. Trying to wean yourself off smoking or nicotine is not quitting in style.

Many so called experts, often entire quit smoking organisations, encourage smokers to cut down rather than quit outright, and offer "support" on the way. The notion that cutting down is an easier or more effective way to quit is false but it is an attractive one to the smoker. It is based on the notion that we smoke or take the drug nicotine at regular intervals out of *habit*, rather than because of addiction, and reflects a widespread ignorance about the addictive nature of nicotine. Based on the idea you need to wean yourself off a useful drug and gradually become accustomed to living without its benefits. Again it's the almost universal assumption that nicotine has beneficial qualities from a drug point of view.

It is not possible to wean yourself off nicotine because it is an addictive substance. When a substance is not addictive you can certainly be weaned off it, for example weaning a baby off milk, where you withdraw the milk for longer and longer intervals. The baby gradually becomes accustomed to not having milk at various times of the day until it eventually gets out of the habit of drinking milk completely.

Retuning to Paracetamol addiction. Imagine you found yourself, for whatever reason, addicted to a drug useless at relaxing you such as Paracetamol, clearly the best remedy would be to throw them in the nearest bin. Would you need "support" to help you through?

You can't just have one. Once you've quit, choosing another cigarette is to choose to return to smoking.

There are absolutely no exceptions. Almost every smoker has quit at some point and then at a later stage attempted to return to smoking as an occasional smoker or lighter smoker. It fails on every occasion. There are no exceptions.

Once you have had even a puff, it is always a slippery slope back to full smoking from that point. Millions of people try and become occasional or light smokers after quitting and every single one of them fails. This is because being a nicotine user, like being a heroin user, is not a habit, it is an addiction. The denial that nicotine is addictive is widespread. When I ask my clients why they smoke, 99% of them say it's out of habit, very few of them even mention the word addiction.

If you have ever played the game Snakes and Ladders you will recall that there are some very long, fearsome snakes near the end of the game, often as you approach 100, that will take you down to near the beginning of the game, say back down to number six or something. Having a smoke or a vape after you have quit is like choosing to go down a snake that actually takes you back down to ZERO, back to the start, back to being a smoker again whatever stage you have got up to when quitting.

This is why nicotine patches, gum and vapes do not work. They do not free anyone from nicotine addiction. All nicotine products do is keep you addicted - every fresh dose of nicotine re-addicts you regardless of how it is administered. Only when a nicotine user stops taking nicotine can they begin to free themselves from nicotine addiction, just like only when an alcoholic stops drinking completely can they free themselves from alcohol addiction.

Once you have broken free from the prison camp of smoking and have made it across enemy lines into to a safe country - never risk going back again. Don't try to sneak back into the camp for a special occasion, like someone's birthday. The gates will close behind you and you will be trapped once again.

Worse still, they will throw you into a more secure unit.

47 - The truth about withdrawal

Most withdrawal is psychological

L ong after physical withdrawal has gone, memories of the pleasure of smoking can still flood into the mind of the former smoker, almost to the point of obsession, especially at times of stress, or in situations where they used to light up. The unenlightened ex-smoker always assumes that this pleasure was brought about by the action of the drug rather than from eliminating withdrawal symptoms. Having no more access to such a "useful" drug they feel deprived. This feeling is termed "psychological withdrawal" and it can be considerably worse and much longer lasting than physical withdrawal. In my opinion it is almost always psychological addiction that causes the nicotine user to cave in and return to smoking or vaping.

Nicotine may be quickly addictive, but it is not deeply addictive like heroin. The true, unavoidable, physical withdrawal symptoms for nicotine are far less severe than most people realise and they start to fade after a week or so. Most of withdrawal is psychological - in other words the belief you've been deprived of a genuinely useful drug. This feeling of being deprived can actually make the physical craving worse and more prolonged. In fact It is the psychological component of this withdrawal that typically exasperates the situation, especially in the longer term. Even when physical withdrawal has ended, the former smoker still feels deprived, frustrated, envious and unhappy.

Compounding this situation is a big surplus of energy that is experienced, especially by heavier smokers, very soon after quitting. Much of what many regard as withdrawal is actually this sudden spike in energy. Smokers, and vape users alike, are used to feeling lethargic or drained, without realising it, because of the constant negative effects of nicotine poisoning.

A smoker is generally less active than a non smoker because of the constant poisoning. On quitting they are suddenly filled with energy levels that they are unused to, which leads to agitation if that surplus energy is not used. This feeling of agitation is actually the body coaxing them to move.

It's rather like when a child is ill in bed and its blood is full of toxins. It's is happy to lie still but as soon as it recovers it finds being made to lie in bed quite agitating and will repeatedly ask to be allowed up. In a similar way, once a smoker quits they are suddenly freed of the normal toxic load they are accustomed to. Like the recovering child, much of the agitation felt is really the body prompting them to move around more. Instead of this many smokers deliberately take it easy after they have quit and actually restrict their more than usual - no wonder they feel agitated.

This is nothing to do with drug withdrawal - and yet withdrawal gets the blame! For this reason it is better to pace around or go for brisk walks when quitting rather than sit still. Smokers often make the mistake of restricting their movements and physical activity while quitting. Some even avoid going out socially for fear of witnessing others smoke outside bars and cafes.

One of the reasons this book is so thorough and repeats the message in so many, various ways is that the understanding that nicotine is a pointless and useless drug must be very deeply entrenched in the mind of the smoker after he or she has quit - especially in testing times.

As long as you are able to recall the message of this book when you have quit, you will find withdrawal, if any, so much easier to ignore. Rather than feeling deprived you will glow with the fact you have given nothing up. Instead you have waked free from an insidious trap.

48 - Tasmanian Flu (Please note - this is an imaginary illness)

Withdrawal isn't that bad - *but feeling deprived is.*

S ome people experience much worse withdrawal than others, but ask yourself, if you were hooked on Paracetamol or Trap-Eze, or any drug you knew to be useless, wouldn't it be a lot easier putting up with the withdrawal, compared to giving up a drug that genuinely did something for you? You wouldn't feel you were depriving yourself of anything at all. Now you have discovered that being hooked on nicotine is as useless as being hooked on one of those drugs you will find that the withdrawal will be much milder or nonexistent, but that doesn't mean there won't be any kind of unpleasantness. So how do you handle it? Most of us have had our fair share of misery and suffering during our lifetimes, but somehow we got through it, like say heartache, an accident, or getting pneumonia.

Imagine a new form of flu sweeps the world and doctors start panicking - let's call it Tasmanian Flu. Scientists predict that millions of people will be killed by the flu, but as so often, they are wrong, and not a single person dies. Not only that, the flu seems to have a remarkable benefit. Anyone who caches it becomes immune to cancer for the rest of their lives. Once the doctors realise this they reverse what they are saying and advise everybody they should do everything they can to catch the flu, in order to become immunised against cancer. Tasmanian Flu is irritating but the symptoms are usually very mild. You get a slight temperature, a dripping nose, and a sore throat but apart from that it is quite bearable and most people can carry on working or even go to the gym.

The following year there is a new epidemic and almost everyone in your town manages to catch the flu. People celebrate as soon as they realise they have Tasmanian Flu, ignoring he irritation, because they know they will be immune to all forms of cancer from then on. Unfortunately you aren't lucky enough to catch it, and so you become one of the few people in your town not to have become immune to cancer. You try getting into close contact with anyone who has the flu, you follow infected people around, you even breathe in sneezes but it's no good, you just don't catch it. Your friends and family all get the flu and are protected, but they are concerned for you, they really don't want you to die of cancer.

Finally they invent a jab that will give anyone the flu on demand. The only problem is it requires a rare ingredient from the Amazon Rain Forest to make it work. Stocks of the jab are running out quickly and a new batch won't be available for years, but luckily your local doctor still has enough to treat about fifty people. You rush to your doctor's and make it just in time before they run out and close the doors. The waiting room is jam packed with others all waiting to be given Tasmanian Flu.

Before the nurse begins giving people the jab the doctor comes out and speaks to the crowd. He reassure everyone that the jab is as harmless as water. A businessman says he has a crucial meeting overseas the next day and expresses concern about the flu symptoms. The doctor reassures him that although they are irritating, the symptoms are relatively mild - a dripping nose, slight temperature, aching limbs, sore throat etc. No one ever gets really ill or dies from it.

He even says you can carry on working or even go jogging. The business man is not impressed. He complains, saying that he usually suffers very badly from flu, much worse that other people. It would be very bad timing for him to go through a week of feeling irritated and the sore throat would ruin his meeting. The doctor looks totally unimpressed, as if the man is a lightweight. The man says he does not like the doctor's attitude, turns round in a huff and leaves, slamming the door.

Next, a well dressed woman objects to the jab, saying she didn't realise you actually had to go through with the flu itself. She had misunderstood and thought it was an inoculation. The doctor explains that you need to go through with the illness in order to become immune to cancer. The woman hesitates, saying it is bad timing, she has booked a box for her friends at the theatre for the following night. She can't bear the thought of going through with the sore throat and the running nose, she hates the idea of feeling irritable for days on end, and says the flu would totally ruin her party. Doesn't he realise she has spent a considerable amount of money on hiring the box? By now, the doctor is getting annoyed. He tells the crowd he is busy and is not interested in hearing about people's minor concerns when after all, the flu will probably save their lives. The woman is furious and leaves the surgery slamming the door even more loudly, so that all the windows shake.

There are no more questions, so the doctor asks who would like to go first. You decide to go for it in style, so you raise your hand and get the jab over with.

The next day you are feeling terrible. Your nose drips, your throat is sore, your body aches and worst of all you have a terrible feeling of emptiness that food and even coffee won't help you with. At work you feel irritated by the slightest thing. Yet, surprisingly you are full of energy and just as the doctor said you find you can go to the gym or even a quick jog. If anything you have more strength and stamina than usual.

That afternoon the irritation increases, and just as you are beginning to feel really sorry for yourself you receive an automatic text from the doctor, informing you that even at this early stage you will already be immune to cancer. The text also gives you details of a long list of other illnesses you are now very unlikely to get. On reading this you punch the air with triumph, and for the rest of the day, despite all the flu symptoms you are smiling constantly. People at work notice you beaming, they look at each other and wonder why you are in such a good mood.

That evening, by coincidence, you have tickets for the same show the woman at the doctor's surgery was going to. Throughout the performance your nose drips, your temperature is high, your throat hurts - you should really be in bed - but you grin and smile throughout the whole thing. You feel like you are floating on air every time you remind yourself you are now immune to cancer. You are so happy you find it easy to concentrate on the show. At funny moments you laugh along with everyone else, even as the catarrh drips down your sore nose. After a while, you do not even notice the flu.

During the interval, the woman in the box sees you coughing and experiencing quite bad flu symptoms. She calls down to you, saying:

"I recognise you. You are one of the fools who took that jab yesterday!" You reply to her: "No, you are the fool for not going through with it!"

It's the same thing with nicotine withdrawal. It may not be nice but just like Tasmanian Flu you can see it as something positive to welcome with open arms. The worst is usually over in under a week, and now you have learnt that nicotine is a useless drug you would be crazy not to go through with it! There will never be a perfect day or perfect time. Regardless of how inconvenient Tasmanian flu is, or how bad it turns out to be, it's worth going through. The same applies to nicotine withdrawal. Every time you remember you have escaped from a drug which is as useless as being hooked on Paracetamol you can celebrate like the man in the theatre. If you are not feeling deprived, when you no longer believe you have given up a useful drug when you quit smoking or vaping, it reduces or evaporates the withdrawal.

In actual fact, a large part of nicotine withdrawal is psychological. That's not to say it isn't real, it's just that the way we view something unpleasant has a remarkable effect of how badly we suffer from it. Nicotine may be quick to get people hooked, but it isn't deeply addictive in the physical way that other drugs like heroin can be, it's actually only a mildly addictive drug.

If you deliberately give yourself Tasmanian flu, any bad feeling that may follow as your friend. Equally, when you quit smoking or vaping, any bad feeling that may follow is your friend, just the same. That's how to see it. That's how to quit.

Regardless of how mild or how bad Tasmanian Flu turned out to be, surely you would choose to go through with it. Surely the best thing to do would be to grin and bear it. We all have to go through a bit of unpleasantness from time to time in our lives, the best way is to do it in style. The best way to quit smoking or vaping is in style!

49 - Willpower

Some people who come to my sessions declare they have no willpower as if they are proud of it. Usually it's an indirect way of laying down a challenge to me, as if they are saying: "If you don't take away my desire to smoke I will use that as an excuse to carry on!

When you think about it, saying "I have no willpower" is like saying "I am weak". It's nonsense because many of the people who say it are tough, successful types, who clearly are not weak at all. When they say they lack willpower it's usually just because they have failed to quit in the past, either because they lacked true motivation, or, much more likely, because they were ignorant of the fact that being a nicotine user is pointless.

One smoker recently told me he had "the willpower of a gnat!" What he was really saying was he couldn't force himself to go through the unpleasantness of nicotine withdrawal. So I pointed out to him that he did have willpower, it's just that he either didn't realise it, or wasn't prepared to use it. After all, some days it can take a massive amount of willpower just to get up in the morning!

Think about it for a minute. You summon up the will to go through the unpleasantness of getting up out of your lovely, warm, cosy bed in order to go to work and earn money, or in order to not let other people down. Sometimes we really, really do not want to get up in the morning! We long to doze and enjoy the golden, sleepy feeling, but if we have a job or need to avoid letting someone down - we get up. It can take a lot of willpower to get up, but we get up. It can be unpleasant, but we get up.

Not only that we do it every day. Day after day!

We are so used to going through that little bit of unpleasantness every day we take it for granted. In fact we are using a lot of willpower to get up but we take it for granted. Most people don't even look upon this as willpower, on account of there being no question of not getting up, saying they have no choice. But actually, we *do* have a choice. We could choose to lose our job or let everyone down.

If you encounter any withdrawal when you quit smoking or vaping it's worth routinely going through any unpleasantness that may come along, just as you routinely get up out of bed every morning. Yes, you have a choice, but remember, smoking is a useless trap.

The way to quit smoking in style is to routinely go through any withdrawal unpleasantness that may come along without even thinking about it, in much the same way you get up in the mornings when you really don't want to. No one is making you get up. For most of us, the main incentive to get up every day is money. No one is making you quit, but the main incentive is not to die. Smoking is not only slowly killing you, every cigarette is aging you, weakening you, and - most ironically of all - nicotine is a totally, utterly and completely useless drug.

Smokers sometimes say to me they wish there was a way they could be forced not to smoke, long enough for them to get over their addiction, like going into nicotine rehab they would consider it.

If you heard on the news that the world's entire nicotine supply had somehow been contaminated with cyanide, and that anybody continuing to smoke or vape would gradually die - that wish would be granted. You wouldn't smoke. Nobody would smoke. Nobody would need any willpower.

Would smokers worldwide then have to go through terrible hardship? I doubt it. They would handle it just like they do when they can't smoke on long haul flights - only this time it would be like a flight o freedom that goes on indefinitely. The mind is quite capable of switching off from smoking. The more unshakeable your determination to never take nicotine again - the more it switches off.

50 - The Myth of the Right Moment

The only time to quit is now - regardless of what is going on in your life. Waiting for the right moment is a myth. There is no right moment. There will never be a right moment!

Imagine you discover that a group of terrorists are considering injuring or killing some of the people in your street. You inform the police who advise all of you to leave the area immediately while they investigate the danger. How long would it be before you got out of town? Minutes? Hours? Days? Weeks? Months? When would be the right moment to quit? Of course you would not hesitate. You would leave straight away. Someone may point out that the terrorists are only *considering* killing you - that nothing is definite - but you would still leave immediately.

The terrorist attacks start and two or three people in your street die - but then there is a lull in deaths and some people decide to stay put. Amazingly, some residents say they are waiting for "the right moment" to leave. Some of those who did actually leave, now return, telling you they were too stressed to stay away, and are not in quite the right frame of mind to leave for good. Others are even going on about how the threat of death is exaggerated.

It's the same with smoking. There is a plot to kill you. Nothing is definite but there is a strong likelihood you will die if you carry on.

For 500 years we have been doing something unnatural - inhaling tobacco, or nicotine vapour, into our lungs. It kills people. Also, the drug nicotine has no benefit and taking it is pointless...so why hang around? There is no right moment to quit. Just quit.

If you discovered that some of your colleagues at work were plotting your murder, how long would it take before you left the company? Would it take you months or years to leave? Of course not. I'll bet you would quit that day, that instant!

QUIT SMOKING (OR VAPING) IN STYLE

Sometimes in life there is no right moment. You decide to leave your girlfriend. You tell a close male friend about your decision, saying you are going to break the news to her the next day, but when you see her you remember it's her birthday. She looks so delighted to see you, and there is so much love in her eyes that you decide to put off telling her for a few days.

Then she suddenly falls ill for two weeks. You don't have the heart to tell her when she is struggling so bravely to get well! The day after she recovers she reminds you that you are about to go on holiday with her - a two week trip you planned for ages that cost you both thousands of pounds. So you decide to tell her when the holiday is over. On holiday you fall and break a leg, but she faithfully nurses you and visits you in hospital every day for a month while your leg is in traction. She is so concerned and caring you feel you cannot tell her you no longer love her until you have returned home and things are back to normal.

By now three months have gone by. You bump into your friend who asks you if you have told her the news yet. You explain to him about putting things off because you haven't found the right moment yet. Your friend is angry with you - telling you that you should just tell her, you agree, but before you know it it's Christmas, and her folks have booked to come over....

Quitting smoking is like ending a relationship. There is no right moment. Life isn't like that. Don't wait for the right moment because it's a myth. It will never come. Just be brave, pick a day and quit.

51 - The Colour of Calm Breathing Exercise

There are moments of stress everyone's lives whether we are smokers or not, for example, setbacks, upsets, conflicts, or worry.

If you should find yourself in a particularly stressful situation while you are going through the quitting process, here is a very easy and effective self hypnosis technique you can use as a coping technique. I have taught this technique to countless people and most of them have found it very useful. You might prefer to refer to it as a breathing exercise, visualisation, NLP or a form of meditation, it doesn't matter what you call it, it will help you calm down and handle whatever is going on around you. Also, if you are unlucky enough to experience any really bad withdrawal pangs, it will help you overcome them, and afterwards you will find it much easier to carry on with everyday life.

So for example, imagine the stress is an argument. All you have to do is retreat from that situation - if possible - and find a place where you can be alone for five minutes or so. It could be a little longer or shorter - there is no exact time. Find a different room if you can, or if you are at home maybe a bedroom - even a bathroom - as long as it's warm and fairly comfortable. As soon as you are there, sit or lie down. Try and relax physically but don't try and block any upset, anger or feelings at first, just give in to however you are feeling, almost as if you were a visitor to your own body, like a curious outside observer. Don't try and change your breathing rate - let it be the way it naturally is. Then focus on the sounds of the world carrying on around you - let them bombard you whether they are soft or loud - surrender to sound. Let the whole world carry on without you for the time being.

Next, leaving your eyes closed. Imagine that the air all around you in the room is beginning to change colour, slowly changing into the colour of calm, whatever you happen to imagine that colour to be. It could be red, orange, pink or blue - whatever colour you like. Imagine the air is slowly getting thicker and thicker with this colour, as if it were like a kind of gas - a wonderful safe, natural calming gas. You can even imagine it coming out of a cylinder in cloud form if you like, and notice how where it comes out of the nozzle, the colour is particularly dense.

It doesn't matter how clearly, if at all, you can visualise this, it is just a non-verbal instruction to your automatic mind, telling it to begin releasing calm. If you can't see the colour in your imagination, think what i would like if you were able to see it.

Allow it to slowly get thicker and thicker all around you, this wonderful, calming, healing gas, and as it gets thicker and thicker the colour gets more and more dense, until it is completely and totally surrounding you.

Once you've imagined that, in your own time, breathe in a deep breath of that wonderful, calm colour right into your lungs and hold it there for a little while. Imagine that all the incredible calm is now being absorbed into your blood and is able to travel to your mind and is being carried to every part of your body calming you right down. Enjoy that for a while, then exhale as soon as holding the breath feels uncomfortable. As you breathe out, if you want, you can imagine you are breathing out a different colour - the colour of stress. Breathe out quickly as you wish, like a dragon breathing out fire - breathe out any tension left in your body. Afterwards, just breathe normally for a while, and enjoy the calm feeling for a bit.

Then, when you are ready, take in another very deep breath of this calm colour, right into your lungs - even deeper. Hold it in your lungs for another five seconds or so, or as long as you wish. Imagine it's being absorbed into your mind and body again, then breathe our any remaining tension.

Finally, take in one last breath of the calm colour, and this time imagine you are able to breathe it right into your head, as if your head were hollow. Imagine the calm colour filling all of your head. This is a powerful signal to your body's own natural ability to release calm.

Once you have exhaled, enjoy the calm for a while, then simply open your eyes and, if you wish, return to whatever situation you were in before the exercise. You will find you are far better able to cope with any stress. Or, you can just enjoy getting on with your ordinary, everyday life.

You can do the exercise several times a day if you want. If the colours that come into your mind vary from time to time, that's fine, just go with whatever colour comes spontaneously.

With practice, you may find you can do the exercise without needing to sit down, or even without closing your eyes. If you are a very good visualiser, you may find you can actually do it in front of people, in secret - without needing to retreat from the stressful situation.

52 - A few Last Tips

Here are a last few tips to help release the power of your mind.

D id you ever see the film "The Matrix" where the heroine Trinity beckons to her group of attackers, as if inviting them to take her on? It's as if she is saying "Come on then, I am not afraid, try me, give it your best!"

Of course we don't all have that kind of strength and courage, but even if there is just a tiny part of you that relishes a challenge, try to release it when you quit smoking. Rise to the challenge and quit with a flourish!

Remember, it's no big deal really. A cigarette is just a stick of dry leaves surrounded by white paper! That's literally all you are up against! People actually put that stick into their mouths and make it into a bonfire by lighting with a flame. Then they inhale the poisonous smoke - with its cargo of nicotine - which is an insecticide.

A vaporiser is an electronic device containing a heating coil that vaporizes an insecticide and delivers it to your lungs with unnatural flavourings and chemicals such as glycerol and propylene glycol.

Once you've quit there is only one cigarette or vape you ever have to avoid... the first one!

How would you resign from a useless job? With a whimper or hesitation? Would you leave with your tail between your legs? Of course not...you would do your best to walk out with an air of confidence and defiance - you'd quit in style. That's exactly how to quit smoking. Walk away without any apology and never look back.

It's much easier to give up something when you know it is useless - so keep in mind as clearly as you can why nicotine is a completely useless and pointless drug. You were addicted to a completely and utterly useless and pointless drug - like being hooked on Paracetamol. Once you have understood this you will find the whole quitting process more of a formality than an ordeal. An easy way to recall why nicotine is useless is to remember one of the crazy stories - the NLP metaphors - like the Strappie Story, Trapeze, or the one about the Rhino. You might as well laugh your way out if the smoking trap.

The physical withdrawal is only very mild - because nicotine is not deeply addictive like heroin. The worst of the suffering is the psychological withdrawal - the terrible feeling of believing you have been deprived of a useful little lift or crutch. It ramps up the physical component, but as long as you understand that you are not being deprived, the psychological addiction dissolves.

The reason so many people fail when they quit isn't because withdrawal is so unbearable, it's that they are not prepared to routinely go through moments of minor unpleasantness. Sometimes people kid themselves they have chosen a bad time to quit. So they decide to give in, return to smoking and wait for a "better time" to come along, maybe when life is less stressful or less demanding. If you encounter any unpleasantness just go through it. If you can't remember how to handle unpleasant moments just remember the Tasmanian flu story.

You can always do the "Colour of Calm" breathing exercise if there is any really bad stress.

If people smoke or vape in front of you - respect their choice to smoke, but remember, they are still in the nicotine trap. They are all slaves to a completely useless stimulant drug. When you watch them repeatedly stubbing out cigarettes again and again, you will never forget the misery of smoking. You will never forget being hooked on something as poisonous and useless, and controlling as nicotine.

Throw away anything to do with nicotine - cigarettes, vapes, tobacco, roll up papers, ash trays, patches, gum, quit smoking drugs....everything. Tell your friends and family you don't smoke. Don't hide the fact you have stopped, be proud of it. If anyone ever offers you a cigarette or a vape, refuse without hesitation or apology. Never apologise for not smoking. Avoid staying too long in smoky environments, as passive smoking can re-addict you just as surely as taking a puff!

You'll still need willpower and determination, but celebrate because you have given nothing up. You have freed yourself from a useless, addictive stimulant that has no benefit, any more than wearing a strappie has any benefit. You are choosing not to end up in the stadium of death. A good choice. Dying from smoking is a pointless death.

There will still be ups and downs in your day as there are in everybody's life, but as a non smoker you are far better able to enjoy all the ups and downs of life - breathing nothing but clear air into your body. You have escaped from a situation as useless as being hooked on Trap-Eze.

Remember, you are an addict. You can't "just have one." By having one you would be going back to smoking or vaping - there are no exceptions because smoking is an addiction and you would simply re-addict yourself. All addicts have to go through the odd moment of unpleasantness to escape and remain free of their addiction. Accept this with open arms, accept it by getting on with your normal life. You have given nothing up, you have made an escape from a useless stimulant drug that has never relaxed anyone, except in the way that Paracetamol relaxes addicts. The pleasure you may remember was actually just the pleasure of coming out of withdrawal for a useless drug that was just a stimulant.

Forget about any failures of the past. If you have tried to quit before and failed - forget about those times. Don't judge yourself by your past. Judge yourself by what you are doing now. You are who you are today. You can stop today. This is your brand new start. Stop making excuses. Just quit. You now know that you are making no sacrifice - so just quit! Not for me, or anyone else, but for yourself. Carrying on with smoking or vaping is like remaining in a comfortable, cosy relationship with someone you know is slowing aging you and killing you, when all you have to do is leave. Just leave and set off on the wonderful road of freedom!

When you are bogged down in a useless, settled relationship, no one else is going to end it for you. Who cares if the new road isn't so cosy at first?

You will be free! Free from the world's most completely and utterly useless recreational drug. Free to breathe in the beautiful clear air of freedom!

Of course you could stay. No one is forcing you to quit! You don't have to leave, you could carry on and stay in a pointless, stinking trap. But why not bravely smile, even if you encounter a bit of difficulty on the journey. Open your arms to whatever comes when you quit - that is how to do it in style! Don't go running back to that stifling relationship every time you feel low or down or upset or stressed. It's like the people who gave up wearing the Strappie, wishing they could go back to wearing the stupid thing and having the unbelievably relaxing, wonderful feeling every time they remove it. They have golden memories of those moments. But wearing the Strappie was pointless. Smoking or vaping is equally pointless.

Sometimes in life you just have to be a little hardship in order to free yourself from something. Once you fully understand why nicotine is useless physical withdrawal often evapourates anyway or becomes much more bearable, and the more you determined you are, the less the hardship becomes.

Be aware that some people never manage to quit - they go on to prematurely age, become ugly, weaken and die at the hands of the world's most useless recreational drug. Worse than being hooked on Paracetamol. Sometimes they only way out of a situation is to accept you're going to need a little but of willpower - like getting out of your warm cosy bed in the morning when alarm goes off. You don't have to, but you do.

Don't listen to people, or politically correct health advisers, who tell you that you may need multiple attempts before you succeed. That's the talk of defeatism. Why quit in a pathetic half measure way? Why listen to people who tell you it's okay to fail?

Actually, smoking is just one big joke! When writing his book I made every effort to avoid it sounding like a lecture or impersonal scientific study. The fact that smokers die needlessly is tragic, the fact that nicotine provides no benefit is tragic, but wherever possible the book tries to drive home each message with as much humour as possible. When smokers realise that despite taking the risks, smoking has never has provided them with any benefit whatsoever they do not know whether to laugh or cry. I believe it's better to laugh. Smoking is a tragedy but it is also just one, ridiculous joke. There is always something to be said for looking at the funny side. If you enjoyed reading any of the crazy stories like The Rhino or Trap-Eze - just try thinking about them when you quit. The best way to quit is to laugh your way out of smoking.

53 - Summary of The Nicotine Trap

Here is a final refresher:

From a drug point of view smoking is just a trap. You get nothing out the first cigarette because you have no nicotine withdrawal to come out of at that stage, however it is a very quickly addictive drug and very soon you become addicted, even though the drug is an unnoticeable, useless stimulant that does nothing for you. Then you are in a trap. The cycle of lighting up to relieve the withdrawal begins. Each time you light up to escape from the withdrawal you are re-addicting yourself with nicotine. This quickly creates a vicious circle and you become a slave to cigarettes.

Gradually you start having to light up more and more often as the withdrawal builds up more quickly and becomes more intense. Soon you are not only smoking every day, you have to light up in the mornings or face having to put up with withdrawal all day long. It continues like this until most people limit it to a packet a day. The longer you go between cigarettes the longer you have to endure the withdrawal. The saddest thing is that most smokers believe that when they light up they are getting the lift from the drug itself, (or at least part of the pleasure), and are completely unaware of the fact that 100% of the pleasure of smoking comes from not from the drug itself, but from coming out of withdrawal for that drug - up to the level that non smokers feel all the time.

54 - Final Word

All you have to do now is pick a time and quit!

The goal of this book has been to enable you to walk free from the smoking trap forever. Any smoker can do it. You can do it. Now you have read the entire book, you should fully understand why nicotine *is* totally and utterly and completely useless from a drug point of view, why smoking has no benefit and why quitting truly involves NO SACRIFICE whatsoever. Most people need to have the truth about nicotine explained to them at some length, either before the penny drops, or they are completely convinced. It isn't because the message is complicated or subtle, it is mainly because it goes against the grain of absolutely everything we have heard, assumed or believed about tobacco and nicotine our entire lives. It's a bit like when you hear an unusual or subtle joke - not everybody gets it straight away.

So when you are ready, throw away everything to do with tobacco or vaping - and quit in style!

Keep the benefits of being a non smoker or non vaper in your mind. You are walking away from playing Russian Roulette with death and illness. You are walking away from premature aging. As you walk into your future as a non smoker you will have far more energy, you'll be healthier, stronger, more powerful and youthful - reaching your full potential as a man or woman. Your skin will look wonderful after a few short weeks. You will feel fantastic about yourself. You will no longer be burning money through burning tobacco or nicotine. You are walking free from a terrible trap. You will no longer be a slave to the world's most useless recreational drug - a stimulant drug that did the opposite to relax you!

And...the greatest benefit of all is that you will become calmer in every situation in your life. The moment you quit a terrible burden is lifted from your life. That burden is dumped behind you into the past where it will remain for ever and ever.

The paradigm shift is only just beginning. Hopefully in a few years time the nicotine user will be a thing of the past.

So don't hesitate...quit in style!

Quit Smoking in Style Group Sessions

If you would like to attend one of Robert's *Quit Smoking in Style* Seminars details can be found online at: http://www.quitsmokingclinic.co.uk

Amazon feedback

If you found his book useful please spread the word through Amazon feedback.

References

Alexandrov. L et al (2016) Mutational signatures associated with tobacco smoking in human cancer. Science. DOI: science.aag0299

Allen, J et al (2016) Flavoring Chemicals in E-Cigarettes: Diacetyl, 2,3-Pentanedione, and Acetoin in a Sample of 51 Products, Including Fruit-, Candy-, and Cocktail-Flavored E-Cigarettes. Environmental Health Perspectives; June 2016 vol124. Issue 6 DOI:10.1289/ehp.1510185

Aubin HJ, et al (2008) Varenicline versus transdermal nicotine patch for smoking cessation: results from a randomized open-label trial, Thorax, August 2008, Volume 63(8), Pages 717-724;

ASH (2015) Local costs of smoking (2015) Action on Smoking and Health, UK

Borland, R. Timea R. Partos, Hua-Hie Yong, K. Michael Cummings, and Andrew Hyland (2012) How much unsuccessful quitting activity is going on among adult smokers? Data from the International Tobacco Control 4-Country cohort survey. Addiction. 2012 Mar; 107(3): 673–682.

Carr, Allen. (2005) "Packing it in the Easy Way" pp.110-116, Penguin, 2005

Carr, Allen. (1995) "The Only Way To Stop Smoking Permanently":page 8, Penguin, 1995

Chapman, S. and MacKenzie, R. (2010) The Global Research Neglect of Unassisted Smoking Cessation: Causes and Consequences. PLoS Med. 2010 Feb; 7(2): e1000216. Published online 2010 Feb 9. doi: 10.1371/journal.pmed.1000216. PMCID: PMC2817714

Dhelaria RK (2012) Effectiveness of varenicline for smoking cessation at 2 urban academic health centers, European Journal of Internal Medicine, July

2012, Volume 23(5), Pages 461-464.

Doran C, Valenti L, Robinson M, Britt H, Mattick R. (2006) Smoking status of Australian general practice patients and their attempts to quit. Addict Behav. 2006 May;31(5):758-66. Epub 2005 Aug 31.Grando, Sergei A. (2014) Connections of nicotine to cancer. Nature Reviews Cancer 14,419–429 (2014)doi:10.1038/nrc3725. Published online 15 May 2014

Hillel Alpert et al (2012) "A Prospective Cohort Study Challenging the Effectiveness of Population-based Medical Intervention for Smoking Cessation," Hillel R. Alpert, Gregory N. Connolly, Lois Biener. Tobacco Control, doi:10.1136/tobaccocontrol-2011-050129

Johnston, Lennox (1952) CURE OF TOBACCO-SMOKING lancet Volume 260, No. 6732, p480–482, 6 September 1952

Johnston, Lennox (1957) The disease of tobacco smoking and its cure - paperback. Christopher Johnson, London.

Kalkhoran, S; Glantz, A (2016) E-cigarettes and smoking cessation in real-world and clinical settings: a systematic review and meta-analysis. The Lancet Volume 4, No. 2, p116–128, February 2016

Morris, Richard et al (2015) "Heavier smoking may lead to a relative increase in waist circumference: evidence for a causal relationship from a Mendelian randomisation meta-analysis. The CARTA consortium." BMJ Open 2015;5:e008808. DOI: 10.1136/bmjopen-2015-008808

Muy-Teck Teh et al (2009) : FOXM1 Upregulation Is an Early Event in Human Squamous Cell Carcinoma and it Is Enhanced by Nicotine during Malignant Transformation; 2009 Plos One Online Journal

Nesbitt P (1969). Smoking, physiological arousal, and emotional response. Unpublished doctoral dissertation, Columbia University.

Olek, Michael J.(2016) "Optimizing natural fertility in couples planning pregnancy." UpToDate. Accessed (Nizard J1. [What Are the

Epidemiological Data on Maternal and Paternal Smoking?]. J Gynecol Obstet Biol Reprod (Paris). 2005 Apr;34 Spec No 1:3S347-52.

Park, S. et al (2014) Clin. Cancer Res. 20, B16; 2014

Parrott, Andy (1998) (Addiction. 1998 Jan;93(1):27-39

Parrott, Andy C. 1999 American Psychologist, Vol 54(10), Oct 1999, 817-820

Pierce, J. and Gilpin, E. (2002) Impact of Over-the-Counter Sales on Effectiveness of Pharmaceutical Aids for Smoking Cessation. JAMA. 2002;288(10):1260-1264. doi:10.1001/jama.288.10.1260

Radford, E. and Hunt, V. Polonium-210: A Volatile Radioelement in Cigarettes.Science 17 Jan 1964: Vol. 143, Issue 3603, pp. 247-249 DOI: 10.1126/science.143.3603.247

Rose et al (2010) -Kinetics of brain nicotine accumulation in dependent and nondependent smokers assessed with PET and cigarettes containing 11C-nicotine. PNAS 2010 107 (11) 5190-5195; published ahead of print March 8, 2010, doi:10.1073/pnas.0909184107

Sanner and Grimsrud (2015) Nicotine: Carcinogenicity and Effects on Response to Cancer Treatment – A Review. Front Oncol. 2015; 5: 196. Published online 2015 Aug 31. doi: 10.3389/fonc.2015.00196 PMCID: PMC4553893

Schane, Rebecca E. (2010) Health Effects of Light and Intermittent Smoking: A Review

Sharma R1, Harlev A2, Agarwal A3, Esteves SC4 (2016) "Cigarette Smoking and Semen Quality: A New Meta-analysis Examining the Effect of the 2010 World Health Organization Laboratory Methods for the Examination of Human Semen." Eur Urol. 2016 Apr 21. pii: S0302-

2838(16)30069-0. doi: 10.1016/j.eururo.2016.04.010. [Epub ahead of print] Tagliacozzo, R and Vaughn, S. (1982) Stress and smoking in hospital nurses. American Journal of Public Health May 1982: Vol. 72, No. 5, pp. 441-448. doi: 10.2105/AJPH.72.5.441

Tsukahara H, et al (2010) A randomized controlled open comparative trial of varenicline vs nicotine patch in adult smokers: efficacy, safety and withdrawal symptoms (the VN-SEESAW study), Circulation Journal, April 2010, Volume 74(4), Pages 771-778

West, Robert (2015) University College London, supported by Cancer Research UK, The National Institute of Health and Care Excellence, the Department of Health, Pfizer and GSK) Smoking in Britain (2015, 3.6) Research Report - How much improvement in mental health can be expected when people stop smoking? Findings from a national survey

Yu et al (2016) Electronic cigarettes induce DNA strand breaks and cell death independently of nicotine in cell lines. Oral Oncology January 2016Volume 52, Pages 58–65

Printed in Poland
by Amazon Fulfillment
Poland Sp. z o.o., Wrocław

18711619R00123